THE
Natural Healing and Nutrition
ANNUAL
1989

THE
Natural Healing and Nutrition
ANNUAL
1989

Edited by MARK BRICKLIN
Editor, *Prevention*® Magazine
and Sharon Stocker Ferguson

Written by the Staff of Rodale Press

Rodale Press, Emmaus, Pennsylvania

"Old-Fashioned, Doctor-Approved Cold Remedies" was adapted from *Cold Cures: The Medical Self-Care Guide to Prevention and Treatment of the Common Cold and Flu,* by Michael Castleman (New York: Ballantine Books, 1987). Reprinted by permission of the author.

"Think It; Heal It!" was adapted from *Who Gets Sick,* by Blair Justice (New York: St. Martin's Press, 1986). Reprinted by permission of the publisher.

The following chapters were adapted from and reprinted by permission of *Medical Self-Care* magazine, P.O. Box 1000, Pt. Reyes, CA 94956 (free sample magazine available on request): "Heart Health Update: Prevention Is Paying Off" ("The Battle for Your Heart," September–October 1987) and "The Yeast Syndrome: Is It for Real?" ("The Yeast Connection," March–April 1988).

Printed in the United States of America on acid-free paper containing a high percentage of recycled fiber.

ISBN   0-87857-807-2   hardcover

2 4 6 8 10 9 7 5 3 1   hardcover

Contents

Nutrition and Health Newsfront

The Healing Power of Nutrition

Protecting and Restoring Your Good Health

Massage Your Mind with Music
The muscles of our brain respond well and willingly to
the ministrations of Paul Horn or Kitaro. . . . .

Peace on the Home Front
Thirty-nine tips from the American Institute of Stress
for making your home a haven instead of a
battlefield. . . . .

Media Madness: Don't Let the News Get You Down
You can develop a healthier response to the daily
barrage of turmoil and tragedy. Here's how. . . . .

Challenge Your Mind and Recharge Your Life
Even monkeys need creative stimulation to be
happy. . . . .

The Healing Power of Walking

Walk for Your Heart's Sake
New studies show lifesaving benefits of regular, take-it-
easy exercise. . . . .

The Exercise/Cancer Connection
Researchers are finding that active people get certain
cancers less often than inactive people. . . . .

Let a Daily Walk Do Your Dieting
Drop 18 pounds without once picking up a calorie
chart. Yes, it's possible. . . . .

Children's Health Updates

SUPPLEMENTS AND COMMON SENSE

Some of the reports in this book give accounts of the professional use of nutritional supplements. While food supplements are in general quite safe, some can be harmful if taken in very large amounts. Be especially careful not to take more than these commonsense limits:

Vitamin A	10,000 I.U.
Vitamin B_6	50 mg.
Vitamin D	400 I.U.
Selenium	100 mcg.

NOTICE

The information and ideas in this book are meant to supplement the care and guidance of your physician, not to replace it. The editor cautions you not to attempt diagnosis or embark upon self-treatment of serious illness without competent professional assistance. An increasing number of physicians are ready to cooperate with clients who want to improve their diet and lifestyle; if you are under professional care or taking medication, we suggest discussing this possibility with your doctor.

Introduction:
How to Get Past
Health Confusion

Have you ever wondered why there is so much confusion—even contradiction—about health ideas?

Now, I'm not even talking about far-out ideas like perfect-health-through-macrobiotics or huge-muscles-through-protein-pumping.

No, I mean the ideas that come from perfectly respectable, even conservative researchers whose work has to be reviewed by a panel of experts before appearing in a scientific journal.

Even from these sources, we often wind up with information that seems to . . . well, wriggle around a bit too much.

It wasn't that long ago that we were all told that polyunsaturated oil was the way to go. That meant corn oil, soy oil, sunflower seed oil. Monounsaturated oil (from peanuts, olives, and avocados, for instance) was said to be either detrimental or neutral. Now the monounsaturates look to be actually *better* for your cholesterol profile.

On the exercise front, it was no more than five years ago that we were told that walking just doesn't measure up. It doesn't raise your pulse high enough, make you huff and puff enough, so it's not aerobic. And aerobic is where it's at—or where it *was*, five years ago. Today, walking has not only caught up with running, it is actually pulling ahead. Seems that not only does it do the job on your heart just as well, it also *doesn't* do a job on your knees at the same time.

There are lots of other examples, many still up in the air. Are a few drinks a day good for your heart? Only a few years ago, the answer was "probably yes." Now, it's "probably no." Or how about a few cups of coffee? The answer to that one is "who knows?" What about aspirin? Same answer.

You could conclude from all this that health—especially

the health-and-diet connection—is not a science at all. Maybe even that the people involved in this research are not as careful as people doing research in chemistry, for instance, where answers seem to stay put a lot longer.

About a decade ago, in fact, someone reviewed a large body of information on health and nutrition and concluded that "facts" in this field have an average half-life of about seven years. That means that after seven years, half the facts you *thought* were facts, are no longer facts. Whether that estimate is accurate or not, I can't say. But there is no doubt that the reliability factor of many health facts fades with time. And so does the confidence we can afford to put in them.

For all of us whose interest in health is practical, this issue can become a major nuisance—if we let it.

What I'd like to do here is to explain why "hard" facts are so rare in health, and what we can do with confidence despite the slipperiness of our information.

Nutrition and health scientists are just as smart as physical scientists. That's not the problem. The problem is *us*.

For starters, all molecules of the same kind—sodium chloride, or salt, for instance—are identical. But we human beings are all different. If you put a certain number of molecule "A" in a test tube with some of molecule "B," you can bet the farm that a certain predictable chemical reaction is going to occur. But if you put a few teaspoons of salt molecules in human beings, some of us will develop high blood pressure and some won't. Why that is so is simply not known.

Some of our differences cluster around obvious traits. Do an experiment on 20-year-olds and you may well get very different results than you will with 80-year-olds.

Do it with women, and you may get very different results than with men.

Do it with people with heart conditions, people on medication, people who exercise daily, vegetarians, or smokers, and you will also likely get results that can't be automatically assumed to apply to all people.

Those are obvious differences. Others aren't so obvious. Let's say you are looking at various health practices in large populations and then associating them with the presence or absence of disease. You may find, for instance, that people who belong to health clubs have a very low rate of heart disease. But before you reach a cause-and-effect conclusion, think about this: People who belong to health clubs *also* smoke less than average, eat healthier food, often take vitamins, tend not to abuse alcohol and drugs, and more. How do you sort all that out? Actually, there are statistical ways of accounting for a few of these things, but when a whole lifestyle is either positive or negative, finding *one* factor that works by itself is awfully difficult.

What gets trickier still is accounting for mental and social factors. People who are better educated, financially well-off, and have good jobs and a happy family life generally have very good health practices. But there is good evidence that the superior health generally enjoyed by that sort of person goes beyond what we would expect, based on those health practices. It seems likely that merely being well educated and enjoying your life confers definite health advantages. Result: more frustration in finding individual practices that promote health.

There's another confounding factor called the Healthy Volunteer Effect. What this means is that whenever you ask for people who want to participate in an experimental health program, you wind up with a group who are going to be healthier than average no matter what you have them do. Their positive attitude, as expressed by their willingness to participate, can be more important than the actual things they do or eat.

On top of that, when people receive a lot of attention, as they do in tests, certain health factors may improve on that basis alone. There's no doubt that people can use the power of their minds to improve their health when they sense they are *expected* to improve. That's called the placebo effect.

There are a zillion other factors. Like:

● Negative placebo power. You don't hear much about this—maybe because I just coined the phrase. It refers to the fact that many people who take something as innocuous as a sugar pill in an experimental setting will develop symptoms ranging from heartburn and itching to headaches, dizziness, and anxiety. Why, no one can say.

● Time of day. Giving a medicine at 10:00 P.M. rather than 9:00 A.M. can produce a strikingly different effect.

● Seasonal differences. Body chemistry can change with weather and climate. So can emotional states.

● Environment. A bug that's going around a laboratory, hospital, dormitory, or neighborhood can make all your subjects sick for reasons unrelated to your experiment.

● Bedside manner. The attitude of the doctor or researcher can influence the outcome. That's true even of lab animals, who may do much better under the care of a gentle technician. One experiment was thrown off because the caretaker played with the animals and stroked them, and their health became much better than it "should" have been.

The Blue-Chip Health Investment System

Now you know why health information can become so tricky. More important, you probably realize that expecting a lifetime guarantee on a "fact" is simply not realistic.

So how do you get past all the confusion?

The method I use is pretty simple. I call it the Blue-Chip Health Investment System, because it's a lot like buying a blue-chip stock.

The appeal of blue-chip stocks—such as IBM, General Motors, and the like—is that there is not *one* reason to buy them but *many.* Typically, such a company has a long record of profit and growth; it has enormous resources and top-notch management, enjoys wide public confidence, and probably manufactures a broad range of products in a field that has a good future. Such a company may have a bad year or two, but over time, its stocks are generally safe and wise investments.

In health, we can do the same thing.

What we do is look for health practices and habits with not one but *many* things to recommend them. And we make them the foundation of our health program.

Here's one example, a recommendation you will come across again and again in this book: Eat lots of fruits and vegetables. Now, let's list the reasons we *now* believe that's a good idea.

Fruits and vegetables:

● Have lots of vitamin C.
● Have lots of beta-carotene, a precursor of vitamin A.
● Have lots of fiber.
● Contain no cholesterol.
● Are nearly all extremely low in fat.
● Are extremely low in saturated fat.
● Are extremely low in sodium.
● Are excellent sources of potassium.
● Are very low in calories.
● Are good sources of trace minerals.

All these things, by the way, are considered to be important in avoiding the most common serious health problems: heart disease, hypertension, stroke, cancer, and obesity.

Now it's possible that *one* of these reasons may be shown in the near future to be false. Maybe even two. Or three! But all *ten?* That's pretty unlikely. Even if half those reasons are wrong, the other five are reason enough to bring home plenty of apples, potatoes, broccoli, melons, and squash.

So you don't need to worry and wonder every time a new nutrition fact is hatched. You've got your own little golden nest egg going.

Another blue-chip health investment I think is worth buying into is walking. Walking looks like it has the power to:

● Help reduce high blood pressure.
● Control or reduce weight.
● Improve your cholesterol profile.
● Prevent osteoporosis.
● Help control blood sugar.
● Strengthen and help the lower back.
● Relax your mind.
● Improve your mood.
● Produce exercise benefits with an extremely low risk of injury.
● Foster longevity.

Again, maybe time will disprove a few of these reasons. But even if half were disproven, the five remaining ones would be reason enough to walk regularly.

A few other blue-chip health practices that quickly come to mind are making whole grains and beans an important part of your diet, drinking plenty of good water, not smoking, and not abusing alcohol.

Besides having multiple justifications, these practices have something else in common: They are all basically natural things for human beings to do. They are part of our heritage, and our bodies seem to thrive on them. The point where natural activities and scientific justification come together is a good starting point for any health program.

Not all basic health practices are purely "natural." Getting regular medical checkups is not exactly an age-old practice, but it makes sense for many reasons. Another blue-chip investment, at least for those who lack a lusty appetite, is a multiple vitamin/mineral supplement: In one fell swoop, you protect against a whole host of potential problems arising from nutritional deficiency.

Think of these investments as the foundation of your health program. Certainly, you can go beyond them—maybe far beyond them. But unless you have a solid base underneath your other health practices, you are not building wisely.

As you read *The Natural Healing and Nutrition Annual* for 1989, keep these thoughts in mind. These new pieces of research must be fitted like stones onto a solid foundation. With that approach, we think you'll find our latest *Annual* not only fascinating but enormously useful as well.

Mark Bricklin, Editor
Prevention® Magazine

Nutrition and Health Newsfront

CHOLESTEROL: SOME CAN CONTROL IT WITH VITAMIN C

Vitamin C packs a one-two punch that may help older people hit cholesterol where it hurts, according to a recent study.

Researchers at the U.S. Department of Agriculture Human Nutrition Research Center on Aging, at Tufts University, studied almost 700 people over age 60. They found that a higher level of vitamin C in the blood correlated with a higher level of high-density lipoprotein (HDL) cholesterol (the protective kind). But the level of total cholesterol was not higher, an indication that low-density lipoprotein (LDL) cholesterol (the kind that blocks arteries) was reduced by vitamin C. (When the researchers checked vitamin C intake instead of blood levels, they found the same effects.) Studies by other researchers with other age groups have shown similar results.

In the Tufts study, the effect of vitamin C was strongest in people between 60 and 69 years old and decreased gradually in older people. The researchers aren't sure why, but they think it may be because the older people had higher HDL levels to begin with.

The researchers estimate that an intake of about one gram (1,000 milligrams) of vitamin C per day could increase

HDL by 8 percent. "Given the magnitude of effect observed in the current report, the potential impact on a large population in terms of [coronary heart disease] is quite significant," they say. "An added benefit is the relative ease and safety with which [vitamin C levels] can be raised" (*Journal of the American College of Nutrition*).

A DOUBLE-BARRELED BLOOD-PRESSURE TREATMENT

A low-sodium, high-potassium diet will usually help lower blood pressure. So will moderate exercise. So perhaps it's no wonder that Florida researchers have found that the two combined lower blood pressure even more.

The researchers studied a group of normal-weight adults with mild hypertension. None were taking blood-pressure medications. After a stabilization period, using a portable blood-pressure monitor at home, half the group went on low-sodium, high-potassium diets. The others followed individually tailored aerobic exercise programs. With either treatment, after about four weeks blood pressure had stabilized at about ten points lower.

Both groups then combined the diet and exercise programs for four more weeks. Their blood pressure dropped an additional four points, putting many of the study's volunteers into the normal range.

"If your doctor clears you for diet or exercise to treat your blood pressure, this study clearly indicates that a combination of the two is more effective than either one alone," says the study's main researcher, James Mitchell, Ph.D. (*Psychosomatic Medicine*).

CAN SCENTS STIMULATE THE IMMUNE SYSTEM?

Imagine the fragrance of a bouquet of flowers or the melody of a favorite song signaling your immune system to fight off cancer. Far out? Researchers at the University of Alabama don't think so.

They found they could "train" the immune systems of mice to rev up when the mice were exposed to an odor. They used a procedure known as classical, or Pavlovian, conditioning. Pavlov, you may recall, conditioned a dog to salivate whenever a bell rang, after learning to associate the sound with food.

The Alabama researchers exposed mice to the odor of camphor for four hours every 3 days for 27 days. Just before being exposed to the smell, the animals were injected with a chemical compound that stimulates interferon. This potent biochemical activates natural killer cells, our body's first line of defense against cancer.

After nine sessions, the rodents were given a three-day rest. On the fourth day, some were exposed to the camphor smell again, but *without* the injection. These mice reacted with three times more interferon production and killer-cell activity than mice that were not exposed.

"We know from studies regarding stress, grief, and happiness that the immune system is linked to the central nervous system," says the research-team organizer. "Now we are beginning to see how we can influence that interaction."

"Our ultimate hope," the researchers say, "is to be able to train the immune systems of people with cancer to mimic the effect of immune-stimulating drugs."

TUMOR SPREAD SLOWED BY FISH OIL

First it was found to fight heart disease, then rheumatoid arthritis, *then* migraine headaches. And now, it seems fish oil can help stop cancer.

In a study by researchers at Harvard Medical School, rats with breast cancers that were known to metastasize, or spread to other parts of the body, were fed one of four diets. They ate either a diet high in saturated fats, one high in polyunsaturated (vegetable) fats, a low-fat diet, or a diet high in omega-3 fatty acids (from fish oil).

Despite their high-fat diet, the rats fed the fish oil survived the longest. At the end of the study period, their tumors were smallest and had spread least.

"It could be that the immune system in animals fed fish oil is better able to recognize tumor cells being foreign, or better able to mobilize its immune system to act against tumor cells," says Debra Szeluga, Ph.D., the study's main researcher.

"I think the evidence suggests that modifying your diet to reduce fat intake and replace red meat with fish would not be an unreasonable thing to do. I think that may help in the prevention, or perhaps even become a part of the treatment, of cancer" (*American Journal of Clinical Nutrition*).

HEAL YOUR HEARTBEAT WITH MAGNESIUM

Heart attack victims who receive a healthy dose of magnesium on admission to the hospital are less likely to suffer dangerous arrhythmias, according to a recent study by Israeli researchers. Such episodes of irregular heartbeat are often a fatal complication of heart attacks.

"Magnesium quickly leaves heart cells after a heart attack. That can cause instability in the electrical properties of the muscles that control the heart's pumping action," says Burton M. Altura, M.D., professor of physiology at the State University of New York Health Science Center in Brooklyn. Raising blood magnesium levels helps to prevent magnesium from leaving heart cells and thus helps the heart endure more stress.

In the study, 48 patients suffering from acute heart attacks received magnesium sulfate as a single intravenous dose. Of those, only 7 went on to develop arrhythmias. Of a group of 46 similar patients receiving a harmless placebo injection, 16 developed arrhythmias (*Archives of Internal Medicine*).

VITAMIN E EASES PMS

Vitamin E has long been a kind of "folk remedy" for premenstrual syndrome. Word that it works spread by word of mouth.

Now a study by Robert London, M.D., of the Johns Hopkins University School of Medicine, supports what some women already swear—that vitamin E relieves PMS symptoms.

In the study, 22 women took 400 international units of vitamin E for three months. Nineteen others took placebos (harmless look-alike pills). All filled out standardized PMS questionnaires at certain times during their menstrual cycle, before, during, and after the study.

The women who took the placebo did find some relief—they had a 14 percent reduction in physical symptoms, such as weight gain and breast tenderness. The women taking the vitamin E, however, had a 33 percent reduction in physical symptoms, a 38 percent reduction in anxiety, and a 27 percent reduction in depression. They were also less tired and had fewer headaches and cravings for sweets.

Why does vitamin E work? Dr. London isn't quite sure. There's some evidence that it can affect the production of prostaglandins, hormonelike substances in the body that may cause some PMS symptoms. Vitamin E is also known to affect neurotransmitters, chemicals that send messages in the brain.

"Our findings should be exciting to the clinician involved in the care of patients complaining of PMS symptoms," he says. "Vitamin E supplementation after appropriate patient evaluation appears to be a rational step in the management of PMS. At the dosage level of 400 international units, no side effects or toxicity was observed" (*Journal of Reproductive Medicine*).

WHAT'S DOWN, DOC?

Scientists have known for some time that carrots can lower cholesterol, but they've only recently confirmed the root cause of this effect.

They knew that certain vegetable fibers have the ability to bind bile acids and lower cholesterol, and they suspected that the two effects were connected. Bile acids are digestive substances in the intestine that are made from cholesterol and are normally reabsorbed after use. But small amounts of them are lost and the body takes cholesterol out of the circulation to make more. So if carrots helped whisk more bile acids out of the body, that could explain their cholesterol-lowering effect.

Peter D. Hoagland, Ph.D., and Philip E. Pfeffer, Ph.D., of the U. S. Department of Agriculture Eastern Regional Research Center in Philadelphia, have found that carrot fiber does indeed bind bile acids. A substance called calcium pectate, a type of pectin, is responsible.

The researchers say that for people with high cholesterol levels, "it may be possible to lower it 10 or 20 percent just by eating two carrots a day." That could be enough to bring many people's levels into the safe range. Incidentally, cabbage and broccoli may produce similar results, the scientists say (*Journal of Agricultural and Food Chemistry*).

B$_6$ DEFICIENCY
CAN HARM COORDINATION

The way you walk may someday be used to spot vitamin B$_6$ deficiency, if preliminary results with laboratory animals hold true for humans. After only nine days on a B$_6$-deficient diet, lab rats began to have subtle problems with the way they moved their hind legs. Those problems were discovered when the rats' footprints were measured. Because rats are biologically similar to humans, there's a good chance that B$_6$ deficiency could cause similar symptoms in humans.

"Ataxia, or loss of coordination, shows up in every species made B$_6$ deficient in experiments—it's universal," explains Monica C. Schaeffer, Ph.D., of the U.S. Department of Agriculture Western Human Nutrition Research Center in San Francisco. "There have also been reports of changes in sensations and sensitivity of peripheral nerves [those that serve the arms and legs]."

What makes Dr. Schaeffer's finding so promising is that the rats were only mildly deficient when they began to have gait problems. "People in this country rarely get severe B$_6$ deficiency," she says. "But food-intake data show that older people and female adolescents often get less than 75 percent of the Recommended Dietary Allowance of B$_6$." Dr. Schaeffer is working to find a test that's sensitive enough to pick up what may be marginal deficiencies.

Good sources of B$_6$ include bananas, vegetables, whole grain products, and meats.

A LITTLE WORKOUT CAN BEAT THE BLAHS

Too tired to wash the dishes, much less stroll around the block? That lack of activity could be causing a vicious circle of fatigue that leaves you too tired for chores—or exercise, says Harold Kohl, a statistician at the Institute for Aerobics Research in Dallas.

Kohl examined the medical charts of patients at the institute. He found the people who complained of chronic fatigue were much less fit and had less stamina than patients who didn't complain of being tired all the time. They did poorly when they were tested on a treadmill. Two years later, though, these same people were much less likely to complain of fatigue if they had improved their cardiovascular fitness through an exercise program. They proved they had become more fit when they were again tested on a treadmill.

"The idea is to make yourself start doing whatever activities you *can* do, however small," Kohl says. "Start a garden. Walk around the block or a mall. Do some housecleaning. You don't have to run a marathon. Just doing a little bit may have obvious energy benefits compared to not doing anything at all."

SELENIUM MAY PUT
SKIN CANCER ON HOLD

Selenium may have the ability to postpone the appearance of skin cancer caused by sun exposure. It may also decrease the incidence of the disease, according to a recent study in laboratory animals.

Karen E. Burke, M.D., Ph.D., of Mount Sinai Hospital in New York, exposed mice to ultraviolet radiation (the component of sunlight that causes skin cancer). Mice that received topical or oral selenium had fewer skin tumors. And the tumors appeared later than in animals not receiving selenium.

What makes this study so exciting is that a special form of selenium applied in a cream worked even better in one breed of mice than selenium added to the drinking water. While the blood levels of the mineral were the same, there was a higher concentration in the skin when the cream was used.

But the cream has other advantages. When sunscreens wash off during a swim, you lose your protection. Not so with the selenium cream. Selenium is absorbed from the cream and stays in the skin.

"The implication is that we now have a cream that could be used as a cosmetic that could stop skin cancer," says Dr. Burke. "Judging from what we're seeing in the mice, we can postulate that the cream could reduce the number of cancers by 40 to 50 percent. And perhaps the onset of cancer could be delayed by five to ten years if children started using it early in life, when they first begin to spend a lot of time in the sun."

That degree of protection could prove especially important if the destruction of the earth's protective ozone layer continues, Dr. Burke says.

This is not the only study to link selenium and skin cancer. In another study, researchers found lower levels of selenium in people who had skin cancer than in people who didn't.

Although Dr. Burke doesn't yet know exactly why selenium has this effect, the prospects are exciting. "We know that selenium prevents cancer by quenching free radicals," says Dr. Burke. "It does this by acting as a cofactor for an enzyme called glutathione peroxidase. But in this study, the levels of that enzyme did not go up. I think we're going to find another role for selenium besides the only one that's known."

HOT PEPPER INGREDIENT HELPS PAIN

People who eat a steady diet of peppery foods usually find that, after a time, they can devour more and more of the hot stuff without feeling the searing effects.

Now researchers have discovered that a drug derived from hot red peppers short-circuits the pain of shingles. A substance in the peppers, capsaicin, depletes a neurochemical that carries pain impulses from the nerves in the skin to the central nervous system. The brain no longer receives pain messages from that area. This same process lets hot-pepper lovers indulge without pain.

Capsaicin is available as an over-the-counter cream, Zostrix. It is also being tested for relieving the pain of mastectomy and diabetic nerve damage.

VITAMIN A HELPS FIGHT KIDS' INFECTIONS

It's not exactly a cure for the common cold. But a group of Australian researchers found that giving vitamin A supplements to preschool-age children who had a history of respiratory infections made a big difference in the youngsters' health. After taking the vitamin, the children had 19 percent fewer respiratory problems than another group of similarly afflicted youngsters.

The scientists at the University of Adelaide prescribed a daily dose of 1,500 international units—well below the U.S. Recommended Daily Allowance. It was administered by the children's parents, who also kept a daily diary of respiratory symptoms during the five-month treatment period and for six months afterward.

Though the vitamin A intake of the supplemented group was much higher than that of the other group, there was no significant increase in their blood levels of the vitamin.

The children who benefited most from the vitamin therapy were those who had a history of lower respiratory illness or allergy (*Australian Paediatric Journal*).

MUSCLE FORCE
MAY MAKE BONES STRONG

Until now, it's been thought that the only exercises to maintain strong bones throughout your lifetime involve weight-bearing activities like running or walking. A new study, though, shows that the most weight*less* exercise of all—swimming—can give similar bone-bolstering benefits.

Researchers at the Portland, Oregon, Veterans Administration Medical Center compared a group of older male swimmers with a similar group of nonexercisers. The swimmers had been doing laps an average of 4.6 hours a week for 13 years.

When the researchers checked the swimmers' spines, they found the vertebrae were 12 percent denser than those of the nonswimmers.

"Contrary to popular belief, it may not be weight bearing but force exerted on the bones by the muscles that's important for increased bone mass," says Eric S. Orwoll, M.D., the study's main researcher. "You can exert a tremendous amount of force on the skeleton by the muscular action of swimming."

And swimming's beauty for people with arthritis, osteoporosis, or other weak spots is that it's relaxing and virtually injury free (*Clinical Research*).

LOWER BLOOD FATS WITH ODORLESS GARLIC

Researchers have long known that raw garlic, eaten in large enough quantities, can reduce harmful blood fats. Unfortunately, people who pursue this treatment develop an odor only another garlic eater could love. What's more, some researchers say that garlic that's "deodorized" by heat treatment has no beneficial effects.

But at least one form of prepared garlic seems to retain its ability to lower blood fats. It's an "odor-modified, cold-aged" product from Japan, called Kyolic.

In a study by researchers at Loma Linda University in California, people with moderately high blood cholesterol added four capsules (one gram) a day of the liquid garlic extract to their regular diet.

For the first few months, their blood fat levels rose—probably as a result of garlic mobilizing body fat stores, the researchers speculate. But then, in most patients, lipid levels dropped, until at six months they were an average of 44 points lower than at the beginning of the study.

"Cholesterol, triglycerides, and low- and very-low-density lipoproteins all dropped, while beneficial high-density lipoproteins rose," says Benjamin Lau, M.D., the study's main researcher. "The garlic seems to inhibit the liver's production of harmful blood fats."

Garlic can't ward off heart disease if you're still eating lots of saturated fats, Dr. Lau says. But if you do adopt a lower-fat diet, it seems that garlic may enhance that diet's artery-cleaning effects (*Nutrition Research*).

CUT YOUR CANCER RISK WITH CAROTENE

A new study has just added to the mounting evidence that people who relish eating fruits and vegetables have a lower risk of lung cancer. And it points to carotene—the form of vitamin A that's found in fruits and vegetables—as the root cause of this reduced risk.

Researchers at the State University of New York at Buffalo compared the diets of 450 people with lung cancer to the diets of more than 900 healthy people. They found that the people with lung cancer had a significantly lower carotene intake than the people without lung cancer. The evidence was strongest in men: Those with the lowest carotene intake had an 80 percent greater risk than those with the highest intake. The effect was greatest in light smokers and those who had never smoked or had quit.

Carotene is converted to vitamin A in the body, and vitamin A is necessary for normal maintenance of epithelial tissues (the type of tissue that lines part of the lungs). That may be why it protects the lungs from cancer, the researchers say. Another possibility is that vitamin A squelches free radicals, compounds in the body thought to instigate cancer.

To see just how much you'd have to change your diet to reduce the risk of cancer, the researchers compared the carotene intakes of those people at highest and lowest risk. The difference in their carotene intakes was about 6,750 international units, the amount of carotene found in a single carrot. "Thus, we can state that dietary modifications to alter one's risk may not require major changes in dietary habits," they say. Their final note: While low carotene intake does increase cancer risk, most lung cancer would never occur if people did not smoke (*American Journal of Epidemiology*).

VITAMINS C AND E AFTER POLYP SURGERY

A new study from Canada shows that supplements of vitamins C and E may help keep polyps of the colon and rectum from recurring. Those polyps are a risk factor for cancer.

Researchers at the Toronto Branch of the Ludwig Institute for Cancer Research gave vitamin supplements to 100 people who had had at least one polyp removed surgically. The supplements provided 400 milligrams of vitamin C and 440 international units of vitamin E daily. One hundred similar patients received a placebo pill (a harmless look-alike).

After two years, the patients were reexamined. Polyps had recurred in 38 percent of the patients who had taken placebos. They recurred in only 30 percent of the patients who had received the vitamin supplements.

"These findings suggest that polyp recurrence may be reduced by about 20 percent with vitamin supplementation," say the researchers. And they say they'd like to see a study with a larger number of people to confirm their findings (*Federation Proceedings*).

A SWEET SOLUTION FOR OBESITY

A natural sugar obtained from fruits, vegetables, and birch bark may someday be used to help people lose weight.

The sugar is called xylitol, and it's commonly used as a sweetener in chewing gum intended for diabetics. But researchers at the Veterans Administration Medical Center in Minneapolis may have found a new use for it.

They found that when a meal contained xylitol, it stayed in the stomach longer. Delayed "gastric emptying" is believed to reduce the total amount of food a person will eat.

To find out if xylitol could do this, the researchers gave volunteers either water, a solution of xylitol, or a solution of another sugar. Then the volunteers were allowed to eat as much as they wanted from an attractive buffet luncheon. The researchers recorded their food intake during the meal.

When the volunteers received plain water prior to the luncheon, they ate an average of 920 calories. But when they received the xylitol solution, they ate only 690 calories at the buffet. In contrast, solutions of other sugars, including glucose, sucrose, and fructose, did not reduce food intake.

"Our data suggest a role for xylitol as a potentially important agent in dietary control," say the researchers (*American Journal of Clinical Nutrition*).

THE LAXATIVE THAT MOVES OUT CHOLESTEROL

An over-the-counter bowel regulator may also regulate cholesterol levels in the people who take it.

In a study by James W. Anderson, M.D., a professor at the University of Kentucky College of Medicine, 26 men with elevated cholesterol levels took either a standard dose of Metamucil or an inactive look-alike three times a day. After eight weeks of treatment, cholesterol levels dropped an average of 15 percent in the men who took Metamucil.

A cholesterol reduction of that magnitude would be enough to bring many people's cholesterol levels into the safe range.

The active ingredient in Metamucil is a plant fiber derived from the husks of psyllium seeds. According to Dr. Anderson, it may lower cholesterol by several mechanisms. One way is by increasing bile-acid excretion. Bile acids are digestive substances that are made from cholesterol and normally are reabsorbed from the intestine after they do their job. But when they're excreted instead, the body has to take cholesterol out of the blood to make more. Psyllium may also slow cholesterol production by the liver, or help the cells eliminate low-density lipoprotein (LDL) cholesterol, the kind thought responsible for clogging arteries.

Dr. Anderson sees Metamucil or other psyllium-seed products as an auxiliary treatment when diet alone doesn't bring blood cholesterol levels down. They may have distinct advantages over potent cholesterol-lowering drugs, which often have undesirable side effects, he says.

Certain high-fiber foods are known to lower cholesterol, too. But a person would have to eat four bowls of oatmeal, two large servings of beans, or four oat-bran muffins a day to get the same amount of fiber the men in the study were taking.

FISH OIL MAY DIMINISH HEART ATTACK DAMAGE

Eating fish oil may actually alter the structure of the heart and protect it from the damage that occurs during a heart attack, according to a new study by researchers at the University of Medicine and Dentistry of New Jersey.

The researchers fed rats diets that replaced vegetable fat with fish oil for one month. They found that the omega-3 fatty acids in fish oil become part of the heart-cell membranes and appear to protect the cells from the damaging effects of reduced blood flow that occurs with a heart attack.

When the researchers induced heart attacks in anesthetized rats that had eaten omega-3 oil, there was very little loss of an enzyme called creatine kinase. Ordinarily, great quantities of this enzyme are lost during a heart attack. The enzyme helps control muscle contraction and thus is vital to heart function.

"We have every reason to believe that similar changes can be produced in humans. Other studies have shown that eating fish or taking fish-oil supplements changes white blood cells and platelets in a similar way," says Carl Hock, Ph.D., the study's director. "Fish oil could help lessen the acute damage that occurs after a heart attack and extend the time available for clot-dissolving therapies to be instituted."

ZINC MAY PREVENT COMMON EYE PROBLEM

Can zinc keep your sight sharp as you age? Now, for the first time, a study from the Louisiana State University Eye Center in New Orleans seems to show it can.

The study included 151 older, healthy people. Half took daily doses of 100 to 200 milligrams of zinc sulfate for 18 to 24 months. The other half took placebos (harmless look-alikes).

Both groups' eyes and vision were checked before and after the study. Researchers looked for "macular degeneration." This is deterioration of vision-forming nerve cells (the retina) in the back of the eye. They found that significantly less loss of vision due to macular degeneration occurred in the zinc takers compared to the other group.

It's not so surprising that zinc worked, says David A. Newsome, M.D., the study's main researcher. "Zinc marshals the function of many important enzymes vital to maintaining normal vision. It's particularly active in the pigmented nerve cells of the retina."

He cautions against taking the large amounts of zinc used in this study without medical supervision. "For right now, I'd tell people to simply try every day to get the Recommended Dietary Allowance—15 milligrams—of zinc." Studies show many people fall seriously short in that regard. Shellfish (especially oysters), meat, liver, and eggs are excellent sources of zinc.

DIABETICS:
RUN TO THE SHOE STORE

The same running shoes that cushion a marathoner's dogs mile after mile might keep a diabetic's feet healthy.

Five to 15 percent of people with diabetes will suffer leg amputation in their lifetime. That's because poor circulation and loss of sensation make their feet vulnerable to infection. Many diabetes-related amputations start with a callus on the sole of the foot that becomes ulcerated and infected. Eventually, gangrene may develop.

And that's where running shoes come in. In a recent study by a Salt Lake City podiatrist, diabetes patients who wore running shoes for 18 months developed many fewer calluses than those patients who did not.

"Most regular shoes, especially those with leather bottoms, do not really cushion the foot," says Scott M. Soulier, D.P.M., of the Utah Diabetes Control Program. "Running shoes are specifically designed with extra cushioning that spreads pressure out over a larger area and helps prevent calluses."

His patients like wearing them, too, he says. "They're a lot more fashionable than custom-made therapeutic shoes" (*Diabetes Educator*).

VITAMINS PRIME ARTERY WALLS FOR HEALTH

When researchers at the University of Mississippi tested the effects of vitamins C and E on atherosclerosis, they weren't too surprised. They had good reason to believe the vitamins would slow down the deterioration of artery walls, and it seems they were right on target.

The researchers fed monkeys a diet spiked with extra cholesterol. Some of the monkeys were given vitamin C supplements, some were given vitamin E supplements, and some were fed a diet with no added cholesterol.

Two years later, the researchers used a technique called ultrasound Doppler analysis to check on two critical measurements of artery disease. One of the measurements is "percent stenosis"—how blocked up the arteries are. The other is "peak velocity"—how fast the blood is moving through the arteries. When arteries are narrowed, the blood must move faster to keep the same amount flowing through. And that's hard on the heart.

The monkeys who took the vitamin supplements had significantly less blockage of their carotid arteries (the ones that bring blood to the brain) than those fed the extra cholesterol without the vitamins. And the peak-velocity measurements were lower in the supplemented monkeys—an indication of less blockage. (The monkeys fed no extra cholesterol fared best of all; they had no blockage whatsoever.)

The researchers decided to try vitamins C and E because they're both antioxidants, substances that protect against the damaging effects of the chemical process called oxidation. But the researchers aren't sure exactly how the two supplements worked. "They may inhibit an enzyme that breaks down artery walls," says Anthony Verlangieri, Ph.D., one of the researchers. "Vitamin E may also interfere with blood clotting." The monkeys were given doses comparable to 2,000 milligrams of vitamin C and 800 international units of vitamin E per day in humans (*Federation Proceedings*).

NUTRITIONAL CATARACT PROTECTION LOOKS GOOD

What you see may depend on what you get in your diet, according to a preliminary study by researchers at the U.S. Department of Agriculture Human Nutrition Research Center on Aging at Tufts University.

They found that people with cataracts had lower levels of carotenoids and vitamin C in their blood than people without cataracts. Carotenoids (beta-carotene and its relatives) are the orange pigments found in carrots, pumpkin, and other vegetables.

Laboratory studies have shown that vitamin C may protect the eye's lenses against the clouding of cataracts. But this is the first evidence that carotenoids may do the same.

The Healing Power of Nutrition

Best Nutritional Bets to Keep Cancer at Bay

Does the word *cancer* scare you? If so, join the crowd.

But how would you feel if you had the nutrition know-how to cut your cancer risk by one-third? Researchers now know that the most common cancers in the United States also have the strongest links with diet, smoking, and drinking. As they're confirming what *causes* cancer, they're discovering what *prevents* it, too.

Out of all this have come dietary guidelines for specific kinds of cancer. Those recommendations are reviewed here, and you'll also read about the most promising new ways to fight cancer with nutrition.

Colon Cancer

Medical researchers have known for some time that there may be several good ways to help prevent this common cancer. Eat more fiber-rich foods, which are believed to dilute any cancer-causing agents formed during digestion. (Most people need to double their fiber intake to reach the recommended 20 to 30 grams a day.) Eat the same bulk-producing bran, whole grains, vegetables, and fruits that relieve constipation. And eat less fat, saturated or otherwise. Keep fat to no more than 30 percent of your calories.

Getting plenty of calcium may be wise, too. Researchers

at New York's Memorial Sloan-Kettering Cancer Center found that 1,250 milligrams a day of calcium slowed the rapid growth of cells lining the bowel. Calcium may neutralize bile acid, which can irritate the bowel and stimulate cell proliferation.

Vitamins E and C also may help neutralize cancer-promoting substances in the bowel. Canadian researchers recently found that when people prone to intestinal polyps took 400 milligrams of vitamin C and 440 international units of vitamin E daily for two years, they developed fewer polyps than those given a nontherapeutic placebo. Polyps are dangerous because they can become cancerous.

And check out beans, rice, potatoes, and seeds. They all contain compounds known as protease inhibitors. In plants, it is widely assumed that these compounds give natural protection against insect predators. In people, they may prove to provide potent cancer protection, says researcher Ann Kennedy, D.Sc., of Harvard University. Protease inhibitors appear to have the talent to make cells revert to normal even after they've already started along the road to cancer, a process known as "initiation."

"Protease inhibitors may be capable of preventing cancer at quite a late stage," Dr. Kennedy says. And even when the protease treatment is stopped, the cells stay normal. They do not return to their precancerous state. Dr. Kennedy does point out, though, that once a cell has become cancerous, protease inhibitors can no longer help.

Protease inhibitors have been found to work in the colon and at several other cancer sites. "There are a number of positive reports on many different organ systems, so it's most likely all kinds of cancer will be affected, except perhaps stomach cancer," Dr. Kennedy says. It is assumed that the stomach's acid content suppresses the action of protease inhibitors.

Dr. Kennedy doesn't know how many cups a day of beans you'll want to eat to stay healthy. But she does offer a suggestion: Try soybeans, the same food she starts with to concoct her laboratory materials. Or try chick-peas. Soybeans have one of the highest concentrations of protease inhibitors of any food, while the protease inhibitors in chick-peas seem to work the best at inhibiting cancer.

Breast Cancer

The key word here is fat. Animals—and people—eating high-fat diets have more breast cancer than those on low-fat diets. Rates are highest in countries where fatty meats and dairy foods crowd the menu. And if you're overweight, your risks increase, too.

Just how fat triggers breast cancer isn't known, says Maureen Henderson, M.D., of the University of Washington in Seattle. It could cause higher levels of hormones that trigger cancer. Calories from other food sources just don't have the same hazardous effects as do fats.

"The standard recommendation is to aim to get no more than 30 percent of your calories from fat," Dr. Henderson says. She is conducting a ten-year-long study to see if a diet containing 20 percent fat fights breast cancer even better. That's about half the fat the average American eats on a daily basis.

There may be a kind of fat you'll *want* to eat if you're concerned about breast cancer. It's the omega-3 oil found in such fish as mackerel, salmon, herring, and tuna. These fish oils block production of potent biochemicals, prostaglandins, which may be involved in cancerous-tissue growth.

One study showed that diets rich in fish oils slowed the growth of transplanted breast tumors in mice. Another showed that breast cancers in rats fed a diet rich in omega-3's grew more slowly and spread less to other parts of the body. In that study, fish oil was better than a low-fat diet at fighting cancer. Substitute fish for meat and you'll be cutting back on your intake of total fat while upping your omega-3's.

Limiting your alcohol intake is also important. Researchers at Harvard Medical School recently found that even as few as three drinks a week put women at higher risk for breast cancer. Women who had one drink or more a day were at 60 percent higher risk than women who did not drink.

Lung Cancer

The best counsel is still this: If you smoke, stop. Get help to stop if you need it.

Until recently, there has been very little nutrition advice

regarding lung cancer. Some studies have shown a protective effect with vitamins C and E. Both these vitamins may help save the lungs from cell-damaging oxidation caused by smoke and air pollution.

More recently, vitamin A and related substances—beta-carotene and retinoids—have moved into the spotlight as lung protectors. Studies have found that blood levels of beta-carotene, and, in some cases, vitamin A, are much lower in the smokers who get lung cancer than in those who don't. Some researchers say that extra beta-carotene in the diet may speed up the normalization of lung tissue in people who have stopped smoking.

Vitamin A and its related compounds are particularly interesting because, like protease inhibitors, they may have the ability to revert cells back to normal even after precancerous changes have occurred. They affect the orderly growth and development of epithelial cells, which line every part of the body from skin to lungs, says Gary E. Goodman, M.D., of the Tumor Institute of the Swedish Hospital in Seattle.

Dr. Goodman is just beginning a study in which smokers and ex-smokers who've puffed the equivalent of a pack a day for 20 years will be given beta-carotene, retinoids or a placebo (harmless look-alike). The beta-carotene group will receive 30 milligrams a day, a superhigh dose that's more than enough to yellow their skin and which requires medical supervision. "There's good reason to think we could see a protective effect," Dr. Goodman says. "But it could be eight to ten years before we're sure of the results of this study."

Folate, part of the B complex, and vitamin B_{12} might also help ex-smokers—and smokers—according to a recent study by researchers at the University of Alabama. They studied smokers with bronchial squamous metaplasia (cell changes that are often considered precancerous). One group of smokers was treated with 10 milligrams of folate and 500 micrograms of vitamin B_{12}. (These amounts far exceed recommended daily allowances and should not be taken without medical supervision.) Another group got placebos. After four months, the supplemented group had significantly fewer precancerous cells than the untreated group.

"Smoking may cause a localized nutrient deficiency in the lungs," says one of the study's researchers. "Adding supplemental folate and related compounds may play a role in preventing cell changes that can lead to cancer. These nutrients may protect the cells' genetic material, chromosomes, from damage by cancer-causing chemicals or viruses."

Mouth and Throat Cancer

These two cancers have a long-accepted link with smoking and drinking. But people with low intake of vitamins A and C also seem to be prone to these cancers. People who get plenty of these nutrients in their diet—through green leafy and yellow vegetables and fruits—may be protected.

Researchers at the Harvard School of Dental Medicine recently found that injections of vitamin E into established tumors in the cheek pouches of hamsters made the tumors degenerate. Vitamin E also induced a large number of cancer-fighting white blood cells to show up on the scene.

The same researchers found that vitamin E completely prevented cancer in hamsters exposed to a cancer-causing agent, and slowed cancer development with even stronger agents. And in another study, supplemental beta-carotene significantly reduced precancerous cell changes in people who chew tobacco.

Researchers have also found that a vitamin A derivative, 13-cis-retinoic acid, given orally, reduced the size of mouth sores in patients with a precancerous condition called leukoplakia. Retinoids could play an important role in oral cancers, these researchers say. They might be particularly important in cases where a cancer is removed, but adjacent, premalignant cells remain, eventually causing a recurrence of cancer.

Cervical Cancer

The thing to remember here is that the cervix is composed of the same sort of cells that make up the linings of the mouth and lungs. So it may be that these cells respond to the same kinds of nutritional deficiencies—or treatments. Studies have found that women with possibly precancerous cervical-cell changes, called dysplasia, or with cervical cancer are more likely to have lower blood levels of vitamin C, beta-carotene, and folate than women without dysplasia.

Studies are currently under way to see if vitamin C helps prevent cervical dysplasia from progressing to cancer. And researchers at the University of Washington plan to give 5 milligrams of folate a day to women with cervical dysplasia to see if it helps to reverse their condition. "A study done several years ago at the University of Alabama indicated that folate does help, but the results were considered controversial," says Joseph Chu, M.D., of the Fred Hutchinson Cancer Research Center, in Seattle. "Researchers do accept the theory that folate might help prevent chromosome damage in cells, but very little is known for sure. It will certainly be interesting to see what we come up with."

Water: A Fountain of Health

By Hans Fisher, Ph.D.

Isn't it amazing how much attention we pay to vitamins and minerals, which are invisible in our food and generally required in such small quantity? By contrast, another nutrient—water—is required in large amounts. Yet most of us pay very little attention to our water needs, even though they are just as critical to our health and well-being. Perhaps because it's so readily available, water is much too often taken for granted.

Life without water is impossible. It is a solvent for most other nutrients. It is a carrier—a waterway from one part of the body to another—for nutrients as well as metabolic waste products. It is necessary as an aid in digestion. And it is a very important factor in the energy and heat balance of our bodies.

When you don't take in enough water, you can be setting the stage for a number of health risks. Water is a detoxifying agent—it literally flushes toxins out of your system. When you don't get enough, toxins can stick around long enough to do damage. Low water intake is also linked to an increased risk of kidney stones. And it's possible that the "shriveled" skin so often seen in older people is not always a consequence of aging but is often due to dehydration.

Adequate intake of water is important because your body is losing water every minute of the day and night. One of the routes for this loss is the air you breathe out. Expired air is always saturated with water vapor, and you may lose half a quart of water per day this way — even when you don't exercise or work strenuously.

You also lose water through your skin — a little more than half a quart a day in a comfortable environment. This loss is called insensible perspiration — you don't even feel it. Insensible perspiration is part of your body's mechanism to maintain and control a constant body temperature.

Water is also lost through excretion. Contrary to what many believe, though, the amount of water lost in the stool is very small (except during a bout of diarrhea). Most of your water losses occur through the urine formed by your kidneys — about 1½ quarts per day.

Getting Enough Water

All of this would be of little concern if we could just "tank up" occasionally and live off the reserve. Unfortunately, we cannot store water in our bodies, so inadequate intake affects us very rapidly. While we can go for relatively long periods of time without food, without water we might only survive for two days in a very hot climate. Luckily, water is usually easy to come by.

We obtain our supply of water from three sources. The most important is the fluid we drink. The second source is the food we eat. Virtually all foods contain some water, and many provide much more than you might think. Meat, for example, can contain 50 percent water or more, and fresh bread may consist of as much as 40 percent. The third source is water formed in our bodies from the metabolism of protein, fat, and carbohydrate. The utilization of 100 calories of carbohydrate provides 15 grams (about one tablespoon) of water; 100 calories of fat, 12 grams of water; and 100 calories of protein, 10 grams.

So how much do you need to come out even? The best estimate suggests that you need about one gram of water for every calorie of energy that you expend. For an average person, that translates into 2 to 3 quarts of water per day. Since you get about 40 percent of that from food and metabolism, the amount you have to drink is roughly 1½ quarts, or six eight-ounce glasses. (If you spend a lot of time outdoors in a hot environment, you'll need even more.)

If that sounds like a lot to you, you're not alone. Most people just don't feel like drinking that much. That's why it's not a good idea to rely on your thirst to guide you. Scientists have recently learned that it's not a good indicator of your need for water.

Special Needs

The elderly and the infirm are highly susceptible to dehydration, so they should take special care to drink enough. Nursing mothers should also be careful to get enough, because studies show that they generally don't drink enough to compensate for the water secreted into their milk.

Athletes need to be especially concerned about their water intake because of the greater amount they lose in perspiration. (In fact, of all the nutrients that have been suggested to improve performance, only water has been shown to be of any meaningful value.)

The high protein intake of most Americans makes adequate water intake even more important. It's needed to help clear the kidneys of protein waste products that can be eliminated only through urine.

How much isn't the only important factor to think about, though. What kind is also a consideration.

Water and Your Heart

Certain minerals are found in our drinking water, and they may contribute appreciably to our intake. Among the more important ones are calcium and magnesium. It's the content of these two minerals that defines water as "hard" or "soft." Hard water has at least 100 milligrams per liter of the compound calcium carbonate, and usually contains magnesium. Soft water has much less calcium and magnesium. But there are other differences as well that might make a big difference to your health.

Some home-use water softeners, for example, replace the high calcium in hard water with sodium. That could cause problems over time, because prolonged high sodium intake has been linked to high blood pressure.

The World Health Organization and the National Academy of Sciences have concluded that there is a relationship between the hardness of our water supply and the incidence of heart disease. Specifically, harder water has been linked to decreased mortality from heart disease.

How does hard water protect your heart? Some studies have shown that dietary calcium might be protective against high blood cholesterol levels and high blood pressure. So hard water, with its high calcium content (as much as 60 milligrams in a quart), might influence the rate of heart disease in that way. But there's another possible explanation. It may not be that hard water is protective but that soft water is detrimental. Because of its low calcium and magnesium content, soft water is more acidic. Toxic metals such as lead and cadmium, which are often present in old iron pipes, are more easily dissolved in it. Those metals may be harmful to the heart.

In any case, if your house does have a water softener, you can avoid the problem: Have a hard-water line connected to your cold-water kitchen faucet and use that as your source of drinking water. If you live in a soft-water area and are concerned about heavy metals, you can install a water filter that removes them, or you can use bottled water.

Calcium:
New Blood-Pressure Buster

Researchers digging into the link between calcium and hypertension are uncovering some odd results. So far, studies show that taking extra calcium may lower blood pressure, raise blood pressure, or have no effect at all! Can't scientists make up their minds?

Actually, such findings make perfect sense, they say. The fact is, different people may respond differently to calcium, just as people with hypertension respond differently to salt. "We know that salt doesn't have any effect on around 40 percent of people with high blood pressure," says prominent calcium-connection researcher Lawrence M. Resnick, M.D., of the New York Hospital-Cornell Medical Center. "This isn't anything controversial, either—it's been known for years. In the same way, we know that calcium is important to some people and not to others."

So, researchers say, the rush is on to further unravel the calcium/hypertension riddle. And so is the push to develop an easy way to tell beforehand if a person's blood pressure will go up or down in response to added calcium.

Here's what the experts know so far—and what they recommend you do about it.

A Simple Little Test

Researchers say that if they can come up with a simple test to identify hypertensive people whom calcium can help, calcium would become a great new alternative to drug therapy for millions of people. Fortunately, they've got some good leads.

"Our studies are narrowing the field of possible mechanisms for such a test," Dr. Resnick says. "Right now we're measuring various hormone levels in the body to try to find changes that occur only in people who respond well to calcium.

"Salt sensitivity in itself also seems to be a key factor. Studies have found that the more that salt is bad for you, the more calcium is good for you," he explains. "They also show that getting extra calcium has no benefit whatsoever if you're not salt sensitive. Young people tend not to be salt sensitive. Blacks and older people are. In general, calcium seems to make a bigger difference as you get older."

Because of this salt/calcium link, a test to detect salt-sensitive people could theoretically also help spot people whose blood pressure dips because of calcium. There is no easy salt-sensitivity test yet, but a few scientists are hard at work on it.

The Right Amount of Calcium

In the meantime, if you're hypertensive, what should you do? Get more calcium in your diet? Less?

"You do what you're supposed to have been doing all along," says Edward Roccella, Ph.D., coordinator of the National High Blood Pressure Education Program for the National Institutes of Health (NIH). "You make sure you get your Recommended Dietary Allowance [RDA] of calcium [800 milligrams per day]. It's not recommended that you 'load up' on calcium to prevent or control hypertension. The research is still incomplete.

"And you have to try to look at calcium in proper context. A person who smokes, is under stress, and is overweight is going to be a lot more at risk for hypertension than someone who doesn't have those controllable risk factors. Someone like that shouldn't think that taking extra calcium will make up for the 20 pounds they should lose or the cigarettes they shouldn't be smoking."

Most researchers agree, including a leading authority on calcium and blood pressure, Norman Kaplan, M.D., from the University of Texas Health Science Center, Southwestern Medical School, in Dallas. "Everyone agrees that there are people out there who will benefit from calcium," he says. "But you have to remember that the studies show that calcium makes some people's blood pressure go up at the same doses that it makes other people's go down. And there are concerns that too much calcium might lead to kidney stones."

Another voice for caution is Roseann Lyle, Ph.D., an assistant professor of health promotion and education at Purdue

University. Her most recent study — published in the *Journal of the American Medical Association* — showed "a modest but significant" drop in blood pressure for a group of men who took 1,500 milligrams of calcium a day in supplement form. (The men all had normal blood pressure to begin with, by the way.)

"Even so, we can't tell people to take excessive amounts of calcium," Dr. Lyle says. "Too much calcium has been proven to cause magnesium deficiencies in animal studies. And we just don't know enough about the long-term effects of high doses of extra calcium in humans. My study showed good results with no side effects over a 12-week period, but what happens after 12 years?

"You can't radically change your intake of a single vitamin or mineral without adjusting the others. So until we have more research, people should simply make sure that they get their calcium RDA," she says.

Get the RDA. Sound advice, but it isn't exactly what you'd call exciting. And besides, after all the publicity on calcium lately, isn't everybody already getting enough of the mineral?

"If our study is any indication, the answer is no," Dr. Lyle says. "We recruited volunteers, and a lot of firemen happened to respond. When we checked the calcium intake of the 75 men we picked for the study, we were surprised to see that only a very small number were getting their RDA!"

Unfortunately, other researchers have also unearthed a lot of possible calcium deficiencies in this country. A massive U.S. Department of Agriculture survey of dietary habits in the United States, for example, revealed that about 80 to 85 percent of women and 50 to 65 percent of men may have been getting less than the RDA of calcium.

So the scientific detective work on the calcium connection will go on. Partly because the stakes are so high.

"About 20 to 25 percent of the population has high blood pressure," says one researcher. "There's a strong desire to find nondrug treatments so that we could avoid having these millions of people on long-term drug therapy. We're desperately looking for ways to lower blood pressure through nutrition."

"We scientists aren't smart enough right now to understand all the subtleties involved here," says Dr. Kaplan. "But we'll figure it out. There are a lot of good studies under way."

If you want to learn more, the National High Blood Pressure Education Program will send you, free of charge, more information about hypertension. Write them at Hypertension Program, P.O. Box 120/80-P, Bethesda, MD 20892.

KEEP YOUR CALCIUM AND MAGNESIUM IN LINE

In a recent study, researchers from several midwestern university and hospital nutrition departments reported that "a majority of the U.S. population consumed less than the recommended amounts of both calcium and magnesium."

They also noted that "the majority of the population groups did not consume appropriate proportions of these two minerals to obtain optimal calcium-to-magnesium ratios." A good ratio, or mix, of the two minerals is thought to help ensure their maximum effect.

What is the optimal ratio? Science hasn't yielded that information yet. But the researchers speculate that you can maintain a proper calcium-magnesium ratio by getting the RDA for each mineral. Ratios (based on 1985 RDAs) for different ages would then be:

- Children aged 1 to 5: 800 milligrams calcium to 200 milligrams magnesium.
- Children aged 6 to 11: 800 milligrams to 250 milligrams.
- Adolescent boys: 1,200 milligrams to 400 milligrams.
- Adolescent girls: 1,200 milligrams to 300 milligrams.
- Adult men: 800 milligrams to 350 milligrams.
- Adult women: 800 milligrams to 300 milligrams.

Update Your Healing Food Knowledge

Eating right is one of the cornerstones of health, because foods have remarkable power not only to nourish us but to help us heal. By now most of us know that the vitamin C in citrus fruits and vegetables is needed by our immune system, that the fiber in fruits, vegetables and whole grains may play a key role in protecting us from colon cancer, and that the calcium in dairy foods can help stave off osteoporosis.

Scientists around the world continue to discover more about the healing role of nutrients. Here are some of the newest findings.

Carrots Help Fight Lung Cancer

When researchers at the State University of New York at Buffalo compared the diets of 450 people with lung cancer to the diets of more than 900 healthy people, they found that those with lung cancer had a significantly lower beta-carotene intake than the healthy group.

In the body, beta-carotene is converted to vitamin A, which is necessary for normal maintenance of epithelial tissue, the type of tissue that lines part of the lungs. This may be the reason that beta-carotene protects the lungs from cancer. Another possibility is that vitamin A inhibits free radicals, compounds in the body that are thought to instigate the onset of cancer.

When the researchers compared the beta-carotene intakes of high-risk people with those of people with the lowest risk of cancer, the difference amounted to about 6,750 international units, the amount provided by a single carrot (*American Journal of Epidemiology*).

Fish Fights on Several Fronts

Researchers here and abroad continue to find ways in which fish and fish oil provide significant health benefits. Here's a rundown on some of these discoveries.

Inhibiting Arterial Plaque ● University of Chicago researchers found the first scientific evidence that fish oil can slow the formation of arterial deposits (plaque). Plaque deposits are the primary cause of heart attacks and strokes. In their study, rhesus monkeys on a diet high in fish oil developed far fewer deposits than monkeys on a diet high in coconut oil. The plaque that did develop in the fish-oil group caused fewer medical complications and contained fewer inflammatory cells. The fish-oil group's levels of low-density lipoprotein (LDL) cholesterol were also lower.

Slowing Cancer's Spread ● In a study by researchers at Harvard Medical School, rats with breast cancers were fed one of four diets: high in saturated fat, high in polyunsaturated fat, low in fat or high in omega-3 fatty acids (fish oil). The rats fed fish oil survived the longest, and at the end of the study, their tumors were smallest and had spread least. Fish oils block production of potent biochemicals, prostaglandins, which may be involved in cancerous-tissue growth. According to Debra Szeluga, Ph.D., the study's main researcher, "Modifying your diet to reduce fat and replace red meat with fish would not be an unreasonable thing to do, especially for breast cancer patients" (*American Journal of Clinical Nutrition*).

Lowering Blood Pressure ● West German researchers at the Central Institute for Cardiovascular Research gave men with mild hypertension two cans of mackerel with tomatoes daily for two weeks. Along with a healthy drop in blood fats, the men's blood pressure dropped significantly. Even when they cut back to three cans of fish a week, their blood pressure remained low until they reverted to eating lots of cold cuts of meat and little fish (*Atherosclerosis*).

Taming Arthritis Pain ● Daily doses of fish oil led to modest but significant improvement in the symptoms of rheumatoid arthritis patients studied at Harvard Medical School and Albany (New York) Medical College. These were the first studies to show definite clinical effects of fish oil on an inflammatory disease.

The cells of the people who ate fish oil were examined to see whether the oil inhibited the generation of inflammatory products, thought to cause or contribute to the painful swelling of arthritis. The fish oil did suppress some of the inflammatory products, and the patients definitely felt better.

"In our studies, the doses were roughly equal to a salmon dinner or a can of sardines," says Joel M. Kremer, M.D., associate professor of medicine at Albany. "We also found benefits four weeks after the fish oil was discontinued," he adds.

Stopping Blood Clots ● Studies have shown that a diet rich in omega-3 fatty acids reduces platelet aggregation. Omega-3's also accumulate in the cells lining the artery walls. These cells make anticlotting prostacyclin, and omega-3's are readily converted into prostacyclin. Both these actions may help prevent heart disease in its early stages.

Mackerel, salmon, trout, tuna, and sardines are richest in omega-3 oils.

Garlic Can Thin Blood

Blood clots are one of the main causes of heart attacks and strokes. Eric Block, Ph.D., professor and chairman of the Department of Chemistry at the State University of New York at Albany, has researched the components in garlic that work specifically as anticlotting agents. The most active ingredient so far is ajoene, which seems to change the surface membrane of platelet cells so they're less likely to stick together. Ajoene may also affect the platelet's ability to produce thromboxane, a chemical that causes clumping.

Right now, the best way to take advantage of garlic's blood-thinning effects is to eat whole bulbs, Dr. Block says.

Low-Fat Dairy Foods Lower Blood Pressure

Two Dutch studies have confirmed the findings of at least three earlier ones. They found that more calcium in the diet correlates with lower blood pressure. In other research by John T. Repke, M.D., assistant professor of gynecology and obstetrics at Johns Hopkins University School of Medicine, pregnant women who took 1,500 milligrams of calcium daily lowered their blood pressure 5 to 6 percent. "Women with high blood pressure can potentially lower it by half," says Dr. Repke. "Although we used supplements for their purity in scientific research, we feel dietary calcium is more important."

Potatoes May Protect against Stroke

A 12-year study of diet and stroke incidence conducted by researchers from the University of California at San Diego School of Medicine and the University of Cambridge School of Medicine in England found that not one stroke-associated death occurred in the people whose diets contained the highest levels of potassium. About a 400-milligram increase in potassium intake was associated with a 40 percent reduction in the risk of stroke-associated mortality. That's roughly the amount in one additional daily serving of a potassium-rich fruit or vegetable (*New England Journal of Medicine*).

One medium potato contains 782 milligrams of potassium. Just don't add salt or boil the potatoes. Salting disturbs our mineral balance and can raise blood pressure, and boiling dissolves up to 30 percent or more of potassium. Instead, steam, bake, or microwave your potatoes.

Other excellent sources of potassium include avocados, raisins, sardines, orange juice, and bananas.

Soybeans and Chick-Peas Offer Potent Cancer Protection

Soybeans have one of the highest concentrations of protease inhibitors of any food. There is some evidence that these compounds may help cells in a precancerous stage revert to normal and that cells stay normal even after the protease treatment is stopped. Once a cell becomes cancerous, however, protease inhibitors can no longer help.

Protease inhibitors have been found to work in the colon and at several other cancer sites (although not in the stomach). Ann Kennedy, D.Sc., a Harvard University researcher, says she can't recommend a specific amount of beans to eat daily. But you can start with soybeans, which Dr. Kennedy uses to concoct her laboratory materials. Or you can try chick-peas, which seem to work the best at inhibiting cancer.

Telephone for Tips on Nutrition

What the heck is a jicama? Can I drink diet sodas if I have high blood pressure? How can I find a nutritionist in town? What foods are rich in zinc?

Those are the kinds of questions fielded every day at nutrition information centers—those food-and-diet "fact banks" that are sprouting up all across the nation.

They are basically nutrition "hotlines" (though in a few cases you can walk in as well as phone in), and more and more people concerned about good food and good health are giving them a ring. They are staffed with people ready to answer your questions, send you brochures and fact sheets, or point you toward some other expert or agency that has the answers if they don't. Usually there is no charge.

Most centers are run by either state departments of health or nutrition departments in universities and hospitals—often paid for by your tax dollars. They are usually staffed by people with master's or doctoral degrees in nutrition, registered dietitians, graduate nutrition students, or any combination thereof. No one knows how many centers there are, though there is probably at least one in every state. (See "How to Find a Nutrition Information Center.")

They are not clinics, so they won't give you tailor-made advice on how you should change your diet, lose 20 pounds, or beat an eating disorder. (If you need that kind of help, the centers tell you to see a physician, nutritionist, or other specialist—and may help you find one close by.) But they can give you loads of general information on just about any topic in nutrition.

Here are some general criteria to help you decide whether the center you've contacted is giving you the most complete information.

● Centers that frequently cite the latest studies are less likely to give you "formula" answers based on dated information. Don't be afraid to ask for complete citations.

HOW TO FIND
A NUTRITION INFORMATION
CENTER

To date, there's no master list or national referral service to help you locate a nutrition center near you. But you can usually get a good lead or two by making a few phone calls to:

• Your County Cooperative Extension Service. Home economists employed by the service can answer your food and diet questions and so act, in effect, as nutrition information centers.

• A registered dietitian (R.D.) or licensed dietitian (L.D.). There's a good chance he or she will know where the nearest nutrition information center is.

• A university's food and nutrition department. If they don't provide a nutrition information service, they may be able to direct you to someone who does.

• Ask the center to translate dietary guidelines into terms that are more meaningful to you. They should be able to tell you, for example, that 1,100 to 3,300 milligrams of sodium is equivalent to about ½ to 1½ teaspoons of salt.

• The best centers take the time to put into perspective the facts you ask for. Our recommendation: Look for a center that not only answers your question but tries to relate that information to the bigger picture.

Nutritionists in the Know

But how good is all this information-for-the-asking? And just how helpful are these centers to people wanting facts they can use? To get an idea, some tough nutrition questions were put to the staff of three top centers.

Good news: The centers got A's for accuracy. For the most part, their answers not only conformed to the best evidence in nutritional research but were usually (not always!) in agreement. The centers differed, though, in their approaches to the answers—in what they thought was important and in how much information they were willing to give.

The three centers queried were the Massachusetts Nutrition Resource Center in Boston, the Penn State Nutrition Center, which is affiliated with Pennsylvania State University, and the Department of Dietetics at Stanford University Hospital, which is affiliated with Stanford University Medical Center in California.

And now the questions.

Can everyone benefit from a low-sodium diet, or just people who are sodium sensitive?

As two of the centers pointed out, sodium is a red-light word for as many as two-thirds of hypertensives (people with high blood pressure) because they're sodium-sensitive—that is, their blood pressure goes down when they decrease their sodium intake. At present, the only way hypertensives can find out if they're among the sodium sensitive is by going on a low-sodium diet and monitoring their blood pressure.

All three centers recommended moderation in salt (sodium) intake, even if you're not hypertensive. But they cited different reasons. Penn State and Massachusetts said you should watch your sodium intake because you probably get far more sodium than your body needs anyway. "The average American diet includes about 5,000 to 7,000 milligrams of sodium per day," Massachusetts said. "The safe and adequate range is between 1,100 and 3,300 milligrams a day." Stanford said you should cut down on sodium because it's part of a healthier eating style. Many high-sodium foods, it pointed out, are also high in fat. And lowering your fat intake is one way to reduce your risk of heart disease.

Does water-packed tuna supply the same level of omega-3 fatty acids as oil-packed tuna?

Though not all the evidence is in yet, all three centers agreed that water-packed tuna probably gives you more omega-3 fatty acids, substances that lower cholesterol and triglycerides and decrease blood clotting. But Penn State provided the clearest explanation why. They pointed out that the oil used in oil-packed tuna is primarily soybean oil, which does *not* provide any omega-3 fatty acids. And since omega-3 fatty acids are fat-soluble, a certain amount leaches out into the vegetable oil. When you drain the oil from oil-packed tuna, 15 to 25 percent of the omega-3 fatty acids are lost, but by discarding the water of water-packed tuna, only 3.1 percent are lost.

Both Penn State and the Massachusetts center went beyond the omega-3 question to say that water-packed tuna also has an advantage in calories and fat. Massachusetts supplied the telling numbers: 100 grams (3.5 ounces) of drained oil-packed tuna deliver a chunky 8.2 grams of fat and 200 calories, while the water-packed variety swims by with only ½ gram of fat and 131 calories.

Do women need to be as concerned about controlling cholesterol levels as men do?

In their own way, all the centers made a case for a resounding yes.

The staff at the Massachusetts center said, "This idea that women are somehow 'safer' arose because in middle age the rates of coronary heart disease for men are three to four times higher than those for women. But coronary heart disease is still the major cause of death in women. And high cholesterol levels are certainly associated with increased risk."

From Penn State, the answer was, "Scientific evidence indicates that elevated cholesterol, along with high blood pressure, smoking, and family history, are the strongest predictors of a person's risk of developing heart disease—in men *and* women."

And Stanford's comments: "Experts say that though women are somewhat protected against heart disease until after menopause, women still need to be concerned about cholesterol and should know what their cholesterol count is."

Are irradiated products on supermarket shelves right now? Are they labeled? Are they safe?

Each center had the facts down pat: Irradiation (which does *not* make food radioactive) involves exposing food to a very short wavelength of radiant energy in the form of gamma rays, x-rays, or electrons. It kills insects, molds and bacteria, extends shelf life, or slows the ripening of produce. Irradiation has been approved by the Food and Drug Administration (FDA) for fruits, vegetables, wheat products, fresh pork, and spices. But the only irradiated products on your supermarket shelves now are a few spices used as ingredients in processed foods. You won't see any labels telling you about the irradiation, though. The FDA doesn't require food manufacturers to list on labels the specific spices used in prepared foods. But a whole jar of spices, a sack of potatoes, a cut of pork, whole fruits and vegetables, a bag of wheat flour—these, if they ever appeared on the shelves, would have to be labeled with words or a symbol to indicate irradiation.

As far as the safety of irradiation is concerned, all the centers were unanimous in their caution, because the issue isn't settled yet. Penn State did the best job of telling why the jury's still out: "Irradiation is a relatively new procedure. Some experts feel that experimental studies to date are sufficient proof of the safety of food irradiation. Other experts feel more conclusive evidence is needed before irradiated foods are considered safe and nontoxic."

Though there was broad agreement on answers here, there were big differences in how each center supplied those answers. The Massachusetts center presented a virtual dissertation, detailing irradiation's history and legal standing, as well as current trends in research. Penn State rendered a much briefer answer but gave references for recent articles on the topic. Stanford did the same and offered to send the latest information on the safety debate.

Is it true that vegetarians can get vitamin B_{12} from tofu, tempeh, and edible seaweed?

All the centers were up on the facts about B_{12} and vegetarians. They supplied plenty of background: Though the vitamin is plentiful in animal foods (such as liver, sardines, oysters, some meats, eggs, cheese, and milk), plants cannot manufacture it. So strict vegetarians (vegans) may have a tough time getting enough B_{12} (even though the Recommended

SIX TOP CENTERS

Here's a directory of a few of the most popular nutrition centers in the country. Three accept inquiries from anyone, anywhere; the rest take calls only from residents of the state in which they operate.

• Nutrition Information Service, Room 101, Webb Building, Birmingham, AL 35294. Services are available to anyone. Call Monday through Friday, 9:00 A.M. to 12:00 noon. From out of state, call (205) 934-3923; Alabama residents call toll-free (800) 231-DIET.

• Stanford University Hospital, Department of Dietetics, Room P1070, Stanford, CA 94305-5223. Services are available to anyone. Call Monday through Friday, 8:00 A.M. to 4:30 P.M. (415) 723-6904.

• Comprehensive Health Education Resource Center, 321 Wallace Ave., Vallejo, CA 94590. Services are for California residents only. Call Monday through Friday, 8:00 A.M. to 5:00 P.M. (707) 557-1592.

• Massachusetts Nutrition Resource Center, 150 Tremont St., Boston, MA 02111. Services for Massachusetts residents only. Call toll-free in Massachusetts: (800) 322-7203, Monday through Friday, 9:00 A.M. to 3:15 P.M.

• Penn State Nutrition Center, Benedict House, University Park, PA 16802. Services are available to anyone. Call Monday through Friday, 8:00 A.M. to 5:00 P.M. (814) 865-6323.

• Nutrition Hotline, Rhode Island Department of Health, Room 302, 75 Davis St., Providence, RI 02908. Services are for Rhode Island residents only. Call toll-free in Rhode Island, Monday through Friday, 9:00 A.M. to 1:00 P.M. (800) 624-2700.

Dietary Allowance is only three micrograms) and may need to find good nonanimal sources to avoid B_{12} deficiency.

All the centers agreed that vegetarians shouldn't count on tofu for B_{12}. Made of soybean curd, this custardlike food has no B_{12} at all.

Tempeh, a fermented soy product, may contain minuscule amounts of B_{12} but should not be considered a good source of the vitamin, the centers agreed. They each explained (with slight differences) why the amount of B_{12} in tempeh is too variable or too low to depend on.

Two of the centers said seaweed isn't a reliable B_{12} source, either. One explained that the B_{12} content varies too much to bank on. The other cited a recent study showing that 80 percent of the B_{12} found in samples of seaweed was B_{12} analogs —forms with no biological value for humans.

True to the principle that simply answering the question is not enough, two centers were quick to mention alternative nonmeat sources of B_{12}. "Nutritional yeast grown on a B_{12}-enriched medium is a reliable nonanimal source," the Massachusetts center said. "Soy milk is fortified with B_{12}, but check the label and choose a brand that gives you a significant amount of B_{12} in a glassful. Also, consider B_{12} supplements."

Nursing the Nervous System with Tryptophan

By Hans Fisher, Ph.D.

Tryptophan has been getting a lot of press recently. Not because it's an essential amino acid from which the body builds protein, or because it's a precursor of the B vitamin niacin. We've known about those functions for years.

The excitement about tryptophan involves things as seemingly diverse as controlling appetite, relieving pain, and getting a good night's sleep. All of these things are affected by the level of serotonin, a chemical messenger in the nervous system. And tryptophan is also a precursor of serotonin.

Scientists are experimenting with tryptophan supplements. They think tryptophan may perform those functions by raising the level of serotonin in the body. Here's what they're finding.

Reducing Weight by Reducing Cravings

People following a very-low-calorie diet often experience a craving for carbohydrates. Drugs that stimulate the release of serotonin by brain nerve cells reduce that craving. Knowing this, researchers at the Obesity Clinic of the University of Lausanne, Switzerland, reasoned that similar results might be obtained if obese people were given tryptophan supplements to raise their brain serotonin levels.

They were right. Moderately obese people who took tryptophan supplements (750 milligrams, twice a day for three months) while on a calorie-restricted diet lost significantly more weight than people who received a placebo (a harmless look-alike).

The researchers speculate that tryptophan might reduce appetite and food intake by increasing the serotonin level in the brain. In severely obese and mildly obese individuals, however, tryptophan had no effect. Even so, the potential of tryptophan supplements in weight loss is so promising that a patent was granted to scientists at the Massachusetts Institute of Technology for a tryptophan-containing supplement for suppressing appetite.

Laying Insomnia to Rest

The evidence indicating that tryptophan helps induce sleep seems incontrovertible. It has been shown to work not only for adults but also for children and even newborn infants. Amounts from as little as 250 milligrams per day have been reported effective in improving sleep in people with insomnia.

In another study by the researchers from Switzerland, people who had suffered from sleeplessness for two or more years slept longer and more deeply after treatment with tryptophan. No changes were observed in a comparison group who received a placebo. The researchers also observed that an increased blood level of tryptophan correlated with an increased duration of sleep.

The most appealing aspect of using tryptophan for the treatment of insomnia is the absence of side effects. It does not cause impairment of reaction time, memory, or motor responses, important factors that can be affected by commonly available sleeping medicines.

Causing Pain to Wane

There is good evidence that serotonin acts as part of the body's defense mechanism against intolerable pain. In one study, cerebral spinal fluid in chronic pain sufferers was found to have no detectable amount of serotonin. People who had no pain had measurable amounts of the neurotransmitter. When tryptophan was given to chronic pain sufferers, they felt significant relief.

In a number of recent studies, it has been found that chronic pain sufferers who take a tryptophan supplement and follow a high-carbohydrate diet have a significant reduction in pain (a high-carbohydrate diet favors an increase in brain tryptophan levels).

In fact, researchers in Italy found that certain drugs that are effective against migraine headaches increase the blood tryptophan level. Researchers theorize that the extra tryptophan is used to make serotonin, which, in turn, provides the relief from migraine pain.

Calming a Movement Disorder

Doctors at the University of Arizona Medical Center recently made an exciting observation. They noticed a reduction in the symptoms of the facial-movement disorder called tardive dyskinesia in a patient who was taking eight grams of tryptophan per day (in four allotments of two grams each). The patient had been suffering from insomnia, and the tryptophan had been prescribed after drugs failed to help relieve the sleeplessness. After several weeks of supplementation, the symptoms of the disorder as well as the insomnia began to improve.

Tardive dyskinesia is brought on by taking certain antidepressant drugs. These drugs have been reported to inhibit serotonin.

In a follow-up study using laboratory animals, tryptophan prevented the onset of tardive dyskinesia when it was given along with an antidepressant drug (haloperidol). Without the tryptophan, the drug did cause the movement disorder.

More Study Needed

Clearly, more study is necessary before these findings can be translated into a meaningful preventive and therapeutic procedure. But tryptophan does look promising.

It's easy to get excited about the potential of tryptophan. But for now, it's important to keep in mind that that's all it is—potential. It would be unwise to experiment on yourself. Instead, seek proper guidance from your doctor in both diagnosis and treatment.

Pack Your Menu with High-Power Nutrition

You try to eat well and make the wisest food choices. But do you have the sneaking suspicion that you could do better, that you could get *more* from your meals if you knew how to combine certain nutrient-rich foods or substitute healthier items for your old standbys? Well, worry no more. Here are 50 ways to boost your food power, along with tasty recipe suggestions to point you in the right direction.

Let Fruit Edge Out Fat ● Make these fruits a low-calorie, low-fat, high-potassium replacement for some of the meat in many recipes. For example:

● Use raisins in a Mexican *picadillo* sauce. Simmer a modest amount of lean ground beef with raisins, chopped onion, chopped tomato, chopped pepper, and chili powder. Use it to fill tortillas or serve over rice or pasta.
● Combine sautéed strips of meat with bananas as they do in many Caribbean and African countries. One suggestion: Marinate lean pork strips in a mixture of stock, ground allspice,

minced garlic, and hot-pepper sauce. Stir-fry with banana coins or spears, and serve over rice.

● When making curries, substitute chopped dried apricots and peaches for part of the meat.

Don't Cook Away Potassium ● Studies suggest that people who eat lots of potassium-rich foods have a reduced risk of strokes. But boiling destroys up to 30 percent of the potassium in vegetables. So either eat your veggies raw or rely more on steaming, microwaving, and stir-frying. Potassium-rich vegetables that microwave well include squash, potatoes, and sweet potatoes. Other high-potassium foods that are excellent microwaved include flounder, salmon, cod, and haddock. Additional ways to increase your potassium intake:

● Toss together a salad of raw spinach, raw julienned beets, sliced apples and sunflower seeds (all decent sources of potassium). Then dress the salad with a vinaigrette made with potassium-rich orange juice.

● Make a quick sauce for fresh fish by combining mashed avocado, chopped tomato, and a dash of hot-pepper sauce.

● Eat more sardines. Add them to green salads, or put them right in your salad dressing: Purée two or three sardines and add to a half cup of vinaigrette. When having a party, serve sardines on an appetizer tray with various mustards, prepared horseradish, and romaine lettuce. To eat, spread a lettuce leaf with mustard or horseradish, top with a sardine and roll up into a cigar shape.

Pit Oat Bran against Cholesterol ● Oat bran is rich in water-soluble fiber, which can help lower cholesterol. To pump up your intake:

● Replace up to half the flour in your favorite muffin recipes with oat bran. Bake as usual.

● Substitute oat bran for two-thirds of the flour in crepe, pancake, and waffle batters.

● Use oat bran instead of flour or bread crumbs to bread chicken, meat, or fish. Season with your favorite herbs.

● Eat cooked oat bran for breakfast. To cut preparation time, use a nine-inch, nonstick skillet instead of a saucepan. The extra surface area allows the cereal to cook faster. Sweeten the cereal with apples, raisins, dried apricots, or prunes.

Look to the Sea for Heart Health ● A diet high in omega-3 fatty acids can help fight heart attacks and strokes. To increase your intake, eat fish frequently. Excellent sources are Norway sardines, salmon, Atlantic mackerel, albacore tuna, sablefish, herring, rainbow trout, and oysters. Here are some interesting ways to include fish in your diet.

● Add a can (3¾ ounces) of drained and mashed sardines to the dough when making soda bread. If your recipe calls for 4 cups of flour, for example, reduce the amount to 3½ cups and mix in the sardines. Bake as usual.

● Braise mackerel with aromatic herbs. Don't skin the mackerel first (the skin will come off more easily after the fish is cooked). Just set one pound of fillets in a large pan in a single layer. Add water to cover, and season with vinegar, garlic, bay leaves, peppercorns, and onion slices. (Or use a combination of lemon juice, garlic, ginger, and chopped scallions.) Cover the pan and either bake for 25 minutes at 400°F or simmer on top of the stove for 15 minutes.

● Microwave one pound of tuna or other fish steaks with chopped tomato, chopped pepper, and hot-pepper sauce. Place in a nine-inch glass pie plate, cover with plastic (leaving one edge turned back for steam to escape), and microwave on full power for about 2 minutes. Then turn over steaks and microwave another 2½ to 4 minutes, or until cooked through. Let stand 4 minutes before serving.

Make the Pectin Connection ● Studies show that this fiber, found in fruits and vegetables, can lower cholesterol. And combining vitamin C with the pectin may reduce it even more. Luckily, many foods high in pectin also contain vitamin C. (Good choices for pectin include soybeans, oranges, pears, potatoes, brussels sprouts, grapefruit, broccoli, tomatoes, spinach, and bananas). Still others can be deliciously teamed with high-C foods.

● Cook dried soybeans until soft, then simmer gently with C-rich green and red peppers, broccoli, or tomatoes.

● Add grapefruit and orange sections to green salads, fruit salads, or chicken salad. Or stew them briefly in apple juice for an unusual compote. For even more pectin, add dried figs and bananas.

● For a new taste treat, eat brussels sprouts raw in salads. Remove the stems and any blemished outer leaves, then thinly slice the sprouts vertically. Toss with red-pepper slivers, chopped broccoli, and red onion. Dress with lemon juice, thyme, and a splash of oil. Serve with poached fish or grilled chicken.

Be a Fiber Finder ● Diets high in fiber have been linked with low rates of heart disease and certain cancers. Boosting fiber can also help you eat less by filling you up sooner. To raise your intake, eat more whole-grain products, fruits and vegetables. For example:

● Add cooked kidney beans to green salads, marinated vegetable salads, and vegetable sautés.

● For a high-fiber, low-fat dessert, serve raspberry cocktail. Fill pretty wine goblets with fresh raspberries, top with thick vanilla yogurt, and garnish with a little grated orange peel.

● Add bran to meat loaves, meatballs, bread dough, and stuffings for fish and poultry. When making stuffing, use three slices of bread and three tablespoons of bran for every four pieces of bread in your recipe.

Pick the Leanest Poultry ● When cooking poultry, remember that some birds are better choices than others. Turkey, chicken, capons, and Cornish hens—all without skin—are much leaner than ducks and geese. And the breast meat is leanest of all. To keep these birds low in fat:

● Poach boneless cuts with chopped tomato, chopped red onion, fresh basil, lemon juice, and water to cover. Serve hot as an entrée or shred for chicken salad.

● Cut boneless breast meat into cubes and toss with lime juice. Sprinkle with oregano and place in a nine-inch glass pie plate. Cover with plastic wrap, turn back one corner for steam to escape, and microwave on full power until pieces are cooked through (stirring at midpoint), about five minutes for a pound of chicken. Toss with a little grated Romano cheese, and let stand for four minutes before serving.

● Thin a bit of coarse mustard with lemon juice, then paint it on Cornish hen halves. Grill over medium-hot coals until cooked through, about 10 to 15 minutes on each side. Remove the skin before eating.

Slash Sodium ● If you're watching your salt intake:

● Create a no-salt seasoning by mashing together one clove of garlic, 1 teaspoon dried sage, ½ teaspoon grated orange peel, and a pinch of ground hot pepper. Use in salad dressings or rub on poultry and meat before grilling.
● Don't automatically salt the water when cooking pasta, rice, and hot cereals. You'll never miss it.
● Check labels on processed foods for sodium content. If nutritional data isn't given, call the Mrs. Dash Sodium Information Center, which can provide sodium figures for many brand-name products plus meats, poultry, fruits, vegetables, and fast-food items. Call (800) 622-DASH (Monday through Friday, 10:00 A.M. to 8:00 P.M. Eastern time).

Feed Your Bones ● To get more bone-building calcium into your diet, feast on low-fat cheeses and other milk products, broccoli, collards, kale, tofu, sardines, and salmon. For example:

● Sauté shredded collard, mustard, and turnip greens with a bit of olive oil and minced garlic. Sprinkle with a little Parmesan cheese and serve hot.
● Mash together canned salmon (bones, too), part-skim ricotta cheese, fresh dill, and snipped chives. Use to stuff tomatoes, peppers, or crepes.
● Use calcium-rich nonfat milk powder in muffins, quick-breads, pancakes, and waffles (add a few tablespoons to each batch). To make skim milk look and taste richer, add two teaspoons of milk powder to each cup.

Fortify Iron with Vitamin C ● Eating vitamin C with iron-rich foods other than meat can help you absorb the iron better. (Good sources of iron include lima beans, sunflower and sesame seeds, soybeans, prunes, raisins, apricots, broccoli, and spinach.) Some easy ideas for pairing the dynamic duo along with these good animal sources of iron:

● Shred cooked turkey meat and toss with orange and grapefruit sections, papaya slices, and a few toasted sunflower seeds. Combine low-fat yogurt with a little thawed orange juice concentrate to use as a dressing. Serve chilled on red lettuce.
● When steaming fish, add chopped tomato and chopped pepper for the last minute or so. Toss with a tiny bit of oil, sesame seeds, and a sprinkle of Parmesan cheese. Serve on shredded spinach.
● Make bean salads with soybeans and Great Northern beans. Combine them with C foods such as broccoli, peppers, and tomatoes.

For Maximum Flavor, Eat Room-Temperature Foods ● Your taste buds can perceive more flavor when foods aren't too cold. So:

● You'll need less dressing on a room-temperature green salad than on a chilled one.
● Grapefruit and other fruit taste sweeter if they're served slightly warm or at room temperature. For a delicious breakfast treat, halve a grapefruit, section it and remove seeds. Then microwave it uncovered on full power until the chill is gone—20 to 30 seconds.
● Poultry salad, tuna salad, and bean salad are more flavorful when the chill is off them. But for safety reasons, don't leave these salads out of the refrigerator for more than 30 minutes—even less in the middle of summer.

Slim Down with Soup ● Starting your meal with a bowl of hot, low-calorie soup can help you fill up so you'll consume fewer calories from your main course than you would otherwise. To keep your soups suitably fit:

● Thicken them with puréed carrots, onions, or spinach instead of butter and flour.
● Make quick soups of leftover vegetables, such as broccoli, carrots, and sweet potatoes. Purée them, then thin with skim

milk. Season the broccoli with grated nutmeg, the carrot with dill, and the sweet potato with orange rind.
● Be sure to degrease your homemade stocks before making soup. The easiest way is to chill the soup overnight. The fat will rise to the top and harden. A superhandy way to remove the fat is with a metal spatula. The fat will adhere to the metal and the soup will drain out through the holes.
● Add onions directly to soups instead of sautéing them in butter first. You'll save both time and calories.

The Healing Power of Vitamin C

Can vitamin C beat the common cold, really? Curb cholesterol? Protect us from the ravages of pollution?

Here's an update on the latest vitamin C research, what scientists are saying about it and where it's headed from here.

Note: The studies discussed in this exclusive report are considered preliminary, but they do emphasize the importance of ensuring that you get adequate amounts of vitamin C (and other nutrients) in the food you eat. To explore the implications of this report further, consult your doctor or a qualified nutritionist.

Cold Facts

The cold war heated up when a new study from the University of Wisconsin's Respiratory Virus Research Laboratory found that vitamin C reduced the severity of the common cold among a few volunteer subjects.

It was only the latest salvo in a does-it-or-doesn't-it controversy that has raged for nearly 20 years since Nobel-prize-winning scientist Linus Pauling urged the use of vitamin C to prevent colds.

Enter Elliot Dick, Ph.D., professor of preventive medicine and director of the Respiratory Virus Research Laboratory at the University of Wisconsin, Madison. Dr. Dick and his fellow researchers selected 16 healthy student volunteers for study. Half received four daily doses of 500 milligrams of ascorbic acid, for a total of 2,000 milligrams daily. The others received a placebo (harmless look-alike). After 3½ weeks of pill swallowing and blood testing, the 16 brave volunteers were housed for a week with eight sneezing sufferers of rhinoviral colds (the rhinovirus is the most common cold virus).

What happened? Seven of the eight volunteers receiving placebos came down with colds, and six of the eight vitamin C takers developed colds. But the colds were much milder among the vitamin C recipients than among the placebo group. The vitamin C group was sick for an average of only 7 days, compared to about 12 days for the non-C group. And the vitamin C group's symptoms during a one-week period were less bothersome. The C group sneezed about 25 times, while the placebo group sneezed about 50; they had fewer than 100 "nose blows," compared to over 125; and they coughed fewer than 400 times, compared to over 1,000.

Dr. Dick says that his study was intended as a better-controlled experiment than those in the past and is hardly the final word. But he notes that public response has been overwhelming. "My major problem is trying to moderate the enthusiasm of others." His researchers are currently repeating the experiment to see if they will produce the same results as before.

He theorizes that if vitamin C can indeed reduce the symptoms of the common cold, it may also reduce its spread. "Mild colds are very difficult to transmit," he says. "This is pretty well understood. So if vitamin C will ameliorate cold symptoms, it may help dampen transmission."

Mystery of the Heart

Can a diet rich in vitamin C increase levels of the "good" high-density lipoprotein (HDL) cholesterol and by doing so reduce the risk of heart disease? That's the question that researchers at the U.S. Department of Agriculture Human Nutrition Research Center on Aging at Tufts University are currently investigating.

The effect of vitamin C on cholesterol has intrigued researchers for more than 30 years. Animal tests first indicated that atherosclerosis can develop when vitamin C intake is very low. Over the next three decades, several more animal and human tests found that the nutrient may affect cholesterol levels, but the results were contradictory.

So for the past five years, researchers at Tufts have methodically undertaken "observational" studies of hundreds of people, looking at their vitamin C intake, total blood cholesterol levels, and HDL cholesterol levels. They haven't found any relationship between C and total cholesterol. But they have found an association between high vitamin C levels in the body and high levels of HDL, which can help keep arteries from clogging.

Their latest study, conducted by Gerard Dallal, Ph.D., and Paul Jacques, Sc.D., found that among 238 elderly Chinese-Americans, those who had high blood levels of vitamin C had higher blood levels of HDL. (This relationship, however, didn't hold true for the smokers in the study.)

The findings were similar to those in an earlier Tufts study of 680 Boston-area men and women over the age of 60. Based on data from that major study, the researchers estimated that people who consumed more than 1,000 milligrams of vitamin C per day had about 8 percent more HDL than those taking less than 120 milligrams daily, and 10 percent more HDL than those taking less than 60 milligrams daily (which is the Recommended Dietary Allowance, or RDA). Although these differences in HDL levels are small, they could be significant in terms of reduced risk of heart disease, the researchers say (*Annals of the New York Academy of Sciences*).

The scientists emphasize, however, that these two studies simply reveal a link between C and HDL—not necessarily a cause-and-effect relationship. The way to find out whether vitamin C is a cause rather than just an innocent bystander is to give people vitamin C and see whether their HDL levels do indeed rise. And that's just what the Tufts researchers have begun to do. "We're giving individuals 1,000 milligrams of vitamin C a day and giving a placebo to a control group," explains Dr. Jacques. The researchers expect to publish results in the future.

In the meantime, it's important to remember the proven ways to reduce risk of heart disease: Quit smoking, cut back on saturated fats, exercise, and shed excess pounds.

Dental Health

If you visit your dentist regularly, brush frequently, floss daily, do everything to the letter of dental law and your gums still bleed, what should you do? First, check with your dentist, because bleeding gums can be a sign of gum disease. And then, dental researchers say, think about whether you're consistently getting enough vitamin C in your diet.

Even in the healthiest mouth, low vitamin C intake may contribute to bleeding gums, says Penelope Leggott, D.D.S., associate professor at the University of California, San Francisco, School of Dentistry. That was what she and researchers at the U.S. Department of Agriculture Western Nutrition Research Center in San Francisco found in a unique, highly controlled study of 11 healthy nonsmoking men who lived at the research center for three months.

All the men had excellent oral health and practiced proper brushing and flossing before and during the study. Their conventional diet was packed with the right amount of nutrients except for one thing: Vitamin C intake varied. For the first two weeks of the study, the men received the RDA of C. For the second four weeks, they got far below the RDA—only 5 milligrams a day. (Although this level was low, it didn't reduce their body stores of vitamin C to scurvy levels.) In the third period, they received ten times the RDA—600 milligrams a day—for three weeks. And finally, there were four more weeks of only 5 milligrams of C per day.

Beginning the second week, the researchers examined the men's teeth and gums weekly—and made some interesting discoveries. First, they found that the intake of vitamin C had no effect on plaque accumulation or on "pocket depths," a measure of the attachment of the gums to the teeth. But one thing did change rapidly during the three-month roller coaster of vitamin C intake: gum bleeding. When the men were at the RDA for C, and during the periods of vitamin C depletion, their gums bled at several sites. The number of sites that bled when probed by a periodontist fell significantly only when the men received amounts of vitamin C well above the RDA (*Journal of Periodontology*).

"These results suggest that under conditions of excellent oral hygiene, proper vitamin C intake may lessen the tendency of the gums to bleed," says Dr. Leggott. "And we also found here that the RDA of 60 milligrams daily may not be adequate under certain circumstances.

"People shouldn't take megadoses, however. If you have an orange, an apple, and a couple of green vegetables every day, you're almost certain to exceed the RDA."

She also warns that vitamin C is not the solution to gum disease: "If people don't brush their teeth, floss, or visit a dentist but take vitamin C, it's not going to help them."

And think twice before trying to get your vitamin C ration from lemon juice, Dr. Leggott says. "I've seen a number of people with very serious etching of their teeth from lemon juice."

Breathing Easier

In one of the newest areas of vitamin research, scientists are investigating ways in which certain nutrients may protect the lungs against air pollutants.

One recent study on the subject comes out of the John B. Pierce Foundation Laboratory at Yale University in New Haven. Researcher Vahid Mohsenin, M.D., conducted a study in which 11 healthy people took either vitamin C (500 milligrams four times a day) or a placebo and then were exposed to either clean air or a small amount of nitrogen dioxide, a pollutant given off by gas appliances and automobile engines. For several days at a time, each person had each of the four possible different exposures: C and clean air, C and nitrogen dioxide, placebo and clean air, and placebo and nitrogen dioxide, in random order.

Dr. Mohsenin found that pretreatment with vitamin C did prevent "airway responsiveness," or irritation. "Nitrogen dioxide causes the airways to become more sensitive," explains Dr. Mohsenin. "Vitamin C basically protected the airways from that state of 'twitchiness.' If subjects didn't take vitamin C and were exposed to nitrogen dioxide, their airways became more irritable," he says.

Dr. Mohsenin says scientists aren't sure yet exactly how

the nutrient might protect the lungs. He speculates that vitamin C might influence levels of prostaglandins or histamines, natural substances that affect responses of muscle tissue in the lung.

"It's too early to say that people should take vitamin C to avoid lung irritation [from air pollution]," says Dr. Mohsenin. "But there are people we measured who had unexpectedly low blood levels of vitamin C. It's possible that people who have lower blood levels of C might benefit from a higher intake, especially if they suffer irritation of the airways as a result of ozone or nitrogen dioxide" (*American Review of Respiratory Disease*).

Fertility Factor

Can vitamin C help build strong sperm six ways? That's what a recent study by scientists at the University of Texas Medical Branch at Galveston suggests. They claim that the study is further evidence of their more than ten years of success in alleviating certain kinds of male infertility with vitamin C.

The head researcher, Earl B. Dawson, Ph.D., associate professor of obstetrics and gynecology at the school, explains that his interest in vitamin C and fertility goes back 20 years. His curiosity was piqued then by studies indicating that the vitamin is essential to the health of the testes and that the sperm of men who were deficient in C showed agglutination— clumping together. Agglutination can cause infertility, says Dawson. "If you have 50 million sperm, and 25 percent are clumped together, there may not be enough 'loose' sperm left to fertilize an egg."

So in 1958 he began recommending vitamin C to would-be fathers. His clinic's standard prescription: 1,000 milligrams a day for ten days, and then 500 milligrams a day for two menstrual cycles.

"This practice has proved successful," says Dr. Dawson. In controlled studies at the clinic, men taking the vitamin C were able to impregnate their wives, while men suffering from the same degree of agglutination who did not take extra C were not.

In the latest study, Dr. Dawson and his colleagues tested the effect of vitamin C on 30 infertile but otherwise healthy men with high agglutination. Some of the men were given 200 milligrams of vitamin C daily; some, 1,000 milligrams daily; and some, a placebo. Every week for three weeks, the researchers measured the men's sperm count (the number of sperm); viability (meaning whether the sperm are alive and moving); motility (forward movement); agglutination; the number of sperm showing abnormalities; and the number that were immature.

The results? The placebo group showed few changes. But after only one week, the 1,000-milligram group showed improvements in all six measures, including a rise of 140 percent in total sperm count. The group taking 200 milligrams, after a week, had improvements that were not quite as dramatic, including a rise of 112 percent in sperm count.

After three weeks, both groups continued to improve. In fact, the 200-milligram men caught up with the 1,000-milligram group, leading the researchers to conclude that the lower dose may be as effective as the higher dose in enhancing fertility (*Annals of the New York Academy of Sciences*).

So should a couple who is having trouble conceiving try vitamin C? "Discuss it with your physician," says Dr. Dawson. "We can't tell everybody who's trying to have a child to try vitamin C—there are so many other factors that should be ruled out first."

But Dr. Dawson does speculate that vitamin C deficiency might be behind as many as 15 percent of the infertility cases in men today.

Update on Fiber and Health

Good health grows on trees! It hangs from apple-laden boughs and courses through crinkly spinach leaves. It hides in carrots beneath the soil and flows in waves of wheat.

And all of this good health is yours for the picking. Because every morsel of food that you get from plants—luscious fruits, crisp vegetables, flavorful grains—contains fiber. And fiber has remarkable power to preserve your health and prevent disease, researchers are finding.

The list of credits so far? Fiber may help prevent heart disease, diabetes, and obesity, research shows. It may even play a role in preventing cancer, some studies suggest. And curing constipation with fiber may be the oldest medical trick in the book.

You may find this all fairly amazing for something often referred to as a "nonnutrient." But the fact is, fiber is the term for the parts of plants that your body can't digest. In most cases, it passes right through your system. But don't be fooled into thinking that fiber doesn't have any effect while it's there.

The first step toward using the health power of fiber is knowing that there are actually several different kinds, each with its own unique ability to keep you well. There's cellulose (the most prevalent fiber, the one that made bran famous), hemicellulose, and lignin, fibers found in whole grains, fruits, vegetables, and beans. There's pectin, the fiber that puts the gel in jelly. And finally, gums, sticky fibers you eat without even realizing it. These plant-derived thickening agents are used in foods as different as bologna and ice cream.

One way to keep all of these straight is to think of them as falling into two categories: insoluble (those that do not dissolve in water) and soluble. The insoluble fibers—cellulose, most kinds of hemicellulose, and lignin—are best known for their ability to ease constipation. The soluble fibers—pectin and gums—are making their name as cholesterol and diabetes fighters. But that's only a small part of the story. For the complete scoop on the most exciting fiber-and-health news, and how-to advice for getting in on a good thing, read on.

Using Fiber to Lower Cholesterol

If you knew that eating lots of delicious fruits and vegetables could lower your risk of heart disease substantially, would you indulge? If your answer is yes, you could be a double winner: You'll get to enjoy those fresh, sweet, juicy, crunchy foods that nature grows and probably lower your cholesterol in the bargain. Water-soluble fibers found abundantly in fruits and vegetables have been shown to lower cholesterol, and that can lower your chances of heart disease.

The fiber called pectin is an old-timer in the ranks of cholesterol fighters. As long ago as 1961, a study showed that eating pectin reduced blood cholesterol significantly. No less than 15 studies have confirmed those early results in the years since. Pectin has the much-sought-after ability to lower low-density lipoprotein (LDL) cholesterol, the undesirable kind, without touching high-density lipoprotein (HDL) cholesterol, the kind thought to be beneficial. What more could you ask?

You could ask that it have a greater effect in the people who need it most—those with extremely elevated cholesterol levels. It does. You could ask that it work together with cholesterol-lowering drugs to bring dangerous levels even lower. It does. You could ask that it work well enough so patients could take less of those drugs and avoid their unpleasant side effects. It does.

Studies have shown that a fiber called guar gum is equally as effective as pectin. And research at the U.S. Department of Agriculture is showing that other gums lower cholesterol, too.

In one study, Kay Behall, Ph.D., a research nutritionist, investigated the effects of three different gums—locust-bean gum, karaya gum, and carboxymethylcellulose—in 12 volunteers. Although they may sound strange, the gums are quite common. Used as thickeners or stabilizers, they are among the top ten ingredients (by bulk) in food production in this country.

The men ate muffins containing one of the gums (in addition to a regular diet) for four weeks. Then they switched to muffins containing the other gums for four weeks each. For the sake of comparison, the men also spent four weeks on a diet with no added gum, and four weeks on a diet with cellulose added instead—a fiber known to have little effect on cholesterol.

The results were similar to those seen with pectin. Total cholesterol was lowered significantly in the weeks that the gums were eaten. Levels dropped from an average of 200 (not very high to begin with) to 170. And as with pectin, HDL cholesterol was unaffected. Cholesterol did not drop during the weeks the men ate cellulose or no added fiber.

In other studies, people with extremely high cholesterol levels saw them reduced after eating foods that included a granola-like bar with either guar gum or locust-bean gum added. They were also able to reduce the amount of cholesterol-lowering drugs they were taking.

While wheat bran doesn't seem to have much effect on cholesterol (it's mostly cellulose), oat bran, with its large proportion of water-soluble gum, can reduce cholesterol levels dramatically. Corn bran falls somewhere in the middle.

What do all of these water-soluble fibers have in common and how do they lower cholesterol? The most important thing seems to be the ability to form a gel with water in the intestines.

Normally, digestive substances called bile acids are secreted into the small intestine following a meal. After they do their job, they're reabsorbed. These bile acids are made from cholesterol. "The feeling is that when you eat water-soluble fibers, such as pectin or gums, bile acids become entrapped in the gel and are carried into the large intestine where they can no longer be reabsorbed," explains Dr. Behall. "The body then has to take cholesterol out of the blood to produce more bile acids. In addition, some of the cholesterol you eat may get caught up in the gel and excreted from the body, too."

Oat bran and dried beans are the only good food sources of gum you can buy at the supermarket right now. The other gums are available only on a commercial basis. Dr. Behall believes that someday they will also be available in the supermarket, baked into granola bars or muffins made specifically for people with elevated cholesterol levels or diabetes.

But pectin is readily available—in fruits and vegetables. Studies show that the amount necessary to lower cholesterol is eight to ten grams a day—the amount in four oranges, for example.

How Fiber Fights Diabetes

In our country, it's fairly common for people over the age of 50 to have some sign of glucose intolerance. This disorder of sugar metabolism often blossoms into type II diabetes, a dangerous disease affecting about 12 million Americans.

The good news is that fiber can help control diabetes, and possibly prevent it in the first place.

The hormone insulin helps your body's cells absorb glucose (sugar), their basic fuel, from the blood. One of the first signs of glucose intolerance is the use of much more insulin than usual to perform this function. The pancreas pours out insulin in an attempt to maintain blood glucose at normal levels, but the insulin receptors in the body's cells appear to become insensitive: They're not getting the message. Eventually, even the high level of insulin secreted can no longer maintain glucose at normal levels and type II (maturity-onset) diabetes develops.

The high levels of insulin bring on even more problems. Insulin is responsible for the efficient conversion to fat of the carbohydrates we eat. When the insulin level is high, the level of triglycerides (a type of blood fat) rises. The level of cholesterol may rise, too. High levels of those two blood fats increase a person's chances of developing heart disease.

That's why the studies linking fiber to better glucose tolerance are so exciting. More than 15 studies in the last ten years show that pectin flattens the rise in blood glucose following a meal. Less glucose in the blood means less insulin needed to bring it down, and triglyceride and cholesterol levels decline. Guar gum also has this effect. And high-complex-carbohydrate, high-fiber diets have been found to help people with type I (juvenile) diabetes as well.

The same property that makes soluble fibers good cholesterol fighters may also make them diabetes fighters: the ability to form a gel.

"It's my opinion that fiber acts primarily to prevent glucose from entering the bloodstream as rapidly as it would if there were no fiber present," says Sheldon Reiser, Ph.D., research biochemist and research leader at the Beltsville Human Nutrition Research Center (BHNRC), a division of the U.S. Department of Agriculture's Agricultural Research Service that is involved in research to determine the best diet for optimum health and well-being.

"[Fiber] forms a gel that acts as a 'diffusion barrier' in the intestine. The glucose has to go through this additional 'membrane' to be absorbed, so it's slowed down," says Dr. Reiser. "The glucose level doesn't rise as fast or as high, and the insulin level doesn't rise as high."

In addition, studies show that the stomach empties more slowly after a meal with lots of fiber. That would slow the absorption of glucose, too.

And a high-fiber diet can help people lose weight. That helps level out glucose peaks and lower triglycerides, because usually, the leaner you are, the more sensitive to insulin your cells become. "It all works together," says Dr. Reiser.

Many studies have shown a significant decrease in blood glucose when ten grams of pectin per day are consumed with meals. The important thing is that it must be present in each meal to have an effect. Fruits, vegetables, oats, and dried beans contain the soluble fiber that helps fight diabetes.

Can Fiber Prevent Cancer?

When studies link fiber with decreased cancer risk, people listen. Of all the nutrients correlated with a decreased cancer risk, though, the argument for fiber is probably the weakest.

"One study that really showed some promising data looked at a very specific type of fiber called pentosans—a type of hemicellulose," says Walter Mertz, M.D., director of the BHNRC. "There was some correlation between the consumption of this fiber and reduced risk for colon cancer. But that's all there is right now."

Drawing conclusions from the research is very difficult because whenever you increase your intake of one thing (fiber), you decrease your intake of something else. Usually, that something else is fat. So which of those changes was responsible for the reduced cancer risk? Studies have shown that people eating diets rich in cruciferous vegetables (broccoli, cabbage, cauliflower) have a lower cancer risk. Is it the fiber or the carotene in those vegetables that's responsible? Or some other component? "It's very difficult to distinguish between these individual influences," says Dr. Mertz. "That's why the whole story is a little bit up in the air right now. We don't have enough data to make a strong statement."

That doesn't mean we should forget about fiber, though. "The fact that this particular aspect is not yet very strong should not deter people from eating fiber," says Dr. Mertz. "Because the recommendation that we should increase our fiber intake is good for many different reasons. I tell people absolutely to continue increasing the amount of fiber-rich foods they eat."

Dr. Reiser agrees. "While the studies do not show definitely that fiber alone reduces cancer risk, they do indicate that a diet that includes fiber reduces the risk. Fiber alone might not do it, but it may be active in combination with other food components." One theory is that because fiber hastens the movement of stool through the intestines, carcinogens (cancer-causing substances) are whisked away before they can do their damage. Another theory is that by increasing the bulk of the stool, fiber dilutes the concentration of carcinogens. The fibers thought to be involved are the insoluble ones and pectin.

Eat More and Lose: Fiber and Obesity

It's a fantasy as old as the hills: to be able to eat as much as you want—even to stuff yourself—without gaining weight. Well, it may not be a fantasy after all, because even if you overindulge in high-fiber foods, you almost can't help but lose. Here's why.

● Most fiber foods are not calorically dense. That means that you can eat an orgy of fruits and vegetables without getting many calories.
● Fiber foods take up a lot of room. You'll feel full on fruits and vegetables before you take in a lot of calories. In one study, people were allowed to eat as much as they pleased with one stipulation. Half the people ate only high-fiber foods. The other half ate only low-fiber, calorically dense foods. The people eating the high-fiber foods were fully satisfied while taking in only *half as many calories* as the people eating their fill of low-fiber foods.

● Fiber foods sneak calories out of your body. In a study by June Kelsay, Ph.D., a research nutritionist at the BHNRC, men on a high-fiber diet excreted 150 calories per day more than men on a low-fiber diet of equal calories. The source of the fiber? Fruits and vegetables.

● Some fiber foods slow down your digestion. When food stays in your stomach longer, you feel full longer.

● Fiber foods have to be chewed well. That gives your body time to get the message that you've had enough to eat. Also, chewing is hard work, so you're likely to eat less.

Fiber Foods Cure Constipation

No argument here. If you have a problem with constipation, adding fiber to your diet will almost certainly help.

Study after study has shown that fiber speeds the movement of stool through the intestines. Why? Fiber has the ability to attract and hold on to water. It makes the stool softer and easier for your intestines to move along.

"It's a very fundamental and simple thing," says Dr. Kelsay. "Yet I don't think there's any question that preventing constipation is important to all of us."

Claims that fiber can prevent hemorrhoids and diverticulitis all center around the ability of fiber to make bowel movements easier. There's no conclusive evidence yet for these claims. But many people find some relief from hemorrhoids with a high-fiber diet.

If constipation is a problem for you, look to the insoluble fibers, cellulose, hemicellulose, and lignin, to do the trick. They're found in whole grains, fruit, vegetables, and dried beans.

Is Fiber Tying Up Your Minerals?

You may have wondered with some concern about reports that fiber interferes with mineral absorption. What's the story?

Some studies have shown that high-fiber foods may decrease the availability of calcium, magnesium, zinc, and iron. There is a problem with the research, though. It's the same problem that plagues the research on fiber and cancer: It's hard to sort out the effects of fiber from the effects of other components in high-fiber foods.

Take wheat bran, for instance. It contains a substance called phytate. There is reason to believe that phytate is responsible for tying up the minerals, or that a combination of fiber and phytate is responsible. In spinach, oxalic acid may be the culprit. In any case, scientists think the responsible parties combine with minerals to make complexes that your body can't absorb.

"There *is* some effect," says Eugene Morris, Ph.D., a research biochemist at the BHNRC. "We're just not sure yet how great it is or exactly what is causing it." Dr. Morris and Dr. Kelsay have done much of the research in this area.

So is this something you should be concerned about? "If you take in too much fiber and too little minerals, it might be a problem," explains Dr. Kelsay. "But there's some suggestion that over a period of time, your body adjusts to this decreased availability. So there is probably no adverse effect even when eating 30 to 35 grams of total dietary fiber a day. It would be hard to eat any more than that because of the volume of food you'd have to consume."

Dr. Morris agrees. "It's my opinion that if you're eating a lot of fiber, you should make sure you're also consuming at least the Recommended Dietary Allowance (RDA) of minerals. If you're getting enough minerals to start with, you're probably safe."

Easing into Eating Fiber

Has the fiber revolution been passing you by? If you're ready to give it a try, you may want to take it easy on your system and get started in a gradual way, because it takes a little while for your innards to adapt to a high-fiber diet. Of course, you won't hurt yourself by jumping right in. It's just that you might feel a little uncomfortable at first ("What's all this rumbling and grumbling in my gut?"), and you don't want to be discouraged right off the bat. So try phasing it in over a week or more, until you find a level that's comfortable for you. And

15 EASY WAYS TO GET MORE FIBER

Now that you know about all of the health benefits of fiber, here are some tips to help you enrich your diet.

1. When you think bread, think brown. Whole wheat (or other whole grain) bread should be the rule, not the exception.

2. Satisfy your sweet tooth with fruit. Berries, apples, bananas, and peaches make excellent desserts.

3. Look for salad bars that offer a wide variety of fresh vegetables—not just lettuce. And make that kind of salad at home.

4. Eat high-fiber cereals regularly for breakfast.

5. Don't peel apples, pears, or peaches when you bake them.

6. Eat potatoes and other vegetables with their skins.

7. Eat vegetables that have edible stems or stalks, such as broccoli.

8. Eat fruits that have edible seeds, such as raspberries, blackberries, and strawberries.

9. Eat dried fruits, such as apricots, prunes, and raisins. Fiber is more concentrated in them (but so are the calories).

10. Eat the membranes that cling to oranges and grapefruit when you peel them.

11. Snack on seeds.

12. Substitute beans for beef in chili or casseroles.

13. Munch on popcorn.

14. Add barley to vegetable soups.

15. Remember that whole grain doesn't have to mean bread or cereal. Try brown rice, corn tortillas, bulgur wheat, or whole wheat pasta.

here's another tip: If you add bran to your diet, drink more water to keep things humming along.

So exactly how much fiber, in grams, do you need? It's a difficult question to answer. For one thing, there are different kinds of fiber. How can you give one number to cover a mixture of entirely different compounds? The optimum range is certainly going to be different for each one. And we don't yet know the optimum amount of each specific fiber. In addition, our methods of analysis haven't been perfected. That also makes it difficult to state exactly how much of each fiber is needed. Finally, people are different, and their fiber needs will probably vary, too.

The studies that have shown the benefits of a high-fiber diet seem to point to a recommendation of 20 to 35 grams per day of "total dietary fiber"—all kinds combined in sort of a lump figure. For practical purposes, a good guesstimate of the optimum amount is up to 30 grams per day.

The best strategy is to eat a wide variety of fiber-containing foods. That way you'll hit on all the different types of fiber and reap all of the benefits that fiber foods have to offer. And you shouldn't have to worry about getting too much fiber—the sheer bulk of the foods will keep you from overdoing it.

Boost Your Daily Energy with a Better Breakfast

Ask a nutritionist what he or she eats for breakfast and you might think you've uncovered a conspiracy. In a survey, the nutritionists questioned listed cereal, cereal and—you guessed it—cereal as their favorite morning food. One might add coffee and orange juice, while another has tea and a sliced banana. But except for weekend extravaganzas, the meal usually centers around a hot or cold whole grain cereal and low-fat milk. That may seem like pretty ordinary fare, but it passes the nutritional test with flying colors. It's fast, light, and right. It actually meets all the requirements of a good breakfast.

And just what is a good breakfast? Nutritionists say it's a meal that provides you with steady energy throughout the morning, keeps you alert but calm, is low in fat and salt and not too high in calories, and helps you watch your weight by taking the edge off what might otherwise be a lunchtime feeding frenzy. A good breakfast is a meal that includes some, but not necessarily a lot, of protein.

In addition to helping your body maintain and repair itself, protein adds an alertness kick to any meal, says Judith

Wurtman, Ph.D., a Massachusetts Institute of Technology research scientist and author of *Managing Your Mind and Mood through Food.* "Protein contains an amino acid called tyrosine," Dr. Wurtman says. "Tyrosine is the major building block from which two major brain chemicals, dopamine and norepinephrine, are made. These chemicals help relay messages through the brain. They help keep you alert and responsive. Getting protein into your system makes your brain able to produce more of these neurochemicals."

The protein in the milk you put on your cereal is enough to get your brain into gear and provides about one-fourth of your day's calcium and vitamin D requirements. You can also get the protein you need from yogurt, cottage cheese, a slice of low-fat cheese, a poached egg, or a piece of fish or chicken.

That milk on your cereal (as well as other protein foods) is a good source of the amino acid tryptophan. Tryptophan is used to produce another important neurochemical called serotonin, which helps people stay calm and focused.

Complex carbohydrates like breads and cereals should also be a big part of your breakfast, nutritionists agree. These starches provide the fuel you need to get your body revved up and going.

If you choose as your complex carbohydrate a whole grain cereal, whole wheat bread, buckwheat pancakes, or waffles, you'll also be taking lots of fiber into your system. Together, complex carbohydrates and fiber help ensure a slow, steady supply of energy throughout the morning, says Brian Morgan, Ph.D., of Columbia University's Institute for Human Nutrition in New York City. "The idea of oatmeal 'sticking to your ribs,' for example, may have some scientific basis in fact. Oatmeal has a nice balance of fibers, which slow the rate at which you digest food. As a result, your blood sugar levels rise slowly, peak later, and stay at a high level longer. You have more energy and can go a long time before you're hungry again." Other low-sugar, whole-grain cereals do the same.

Eat Breakfast to Lose Weight

Skipping breakfast almost always backfires on people trying to diet. Their early-morning good intentions leave them so ravenous later in the day that they'll eat anything that can't escape. They're so hungry their will power disappears.

And their late-afternoon and evening overload means they are taking in calories at a time when their bodies are most likely to store them as fat. Calories eaten early in the day, when people are physically active, are burned up as fuel faster than evening repasts.

You don't need to get a lot of calories at breakfast, but you should eat enough to satisfy your hunger. That might be somewhere between 200 and 500 calories.

"But I'm Not Hungry!"

You say the thought of eating breakfast leaves you cold? See if your morning appetite perks up when you forgo those pound-producing late-evening cookie-eating contests. Start out slow. Try a piece of toast or a small bowl of cereal.

And you don't have to eat the instant you pop out of bed, either. If you need to be up and around for an hour or two before breakfast becomes appealing, that's fine.

"The time of morning that you eat really doesn't matter," Dr. Morgan says. "But people who don't eat breakfast tend to start feeling tired and dull around 11 o'clock, so they will want to eat by then." Brown-bag a breakfast to work, or pick up yogurt, fruit, a little box of dry cereal and a container of milk, or even a sandwich.

A Kick from Caffeine

As most coffee drinkers are aware, their favorite beverage has a beneficial effect on their mental processes, especially coffee drunk first thing in the morning. As a client of Dr. Wurtman's put it, "That first cup of the day seems to clear the cobwebs from the brain."

In fact, researchers at the Massachusetts Institute of Technology have demonstrated the effects of caffeine on cerebral activity. On days when a volunteer took a caffeine pill, he or she consistently demonstrated increased reaction speed, better concentration, and greater accuracy than on caffeine-free days. The results were particularly interesting in an hour-long "vigilance test" where volunteers had to recognize and respond to a series of tones. Volunteers who had taken a caffeine pill remained alert and attentive to the end of the test, Dr. Wurtman says. "But when those same volunteers were given a placebo, they became restless and bored. Some simply tuned out, and a few went to sleep." The caffeine worked equally well on people who normally *never* drank coffee.

For those who feel they need the boost, Dr. Wurtman suggests, "To start the day in top mental form, drink one or two cups of coffee soon after you get out of bed." Of course, if you're the type who becomes jittery from caffeine, you'll want to steer clear of even this small amount.

Midmorning Reinforcements

If you rise and eat very early, or if you know you perform better with mini-meals throughout the day, you may want to save part of your breakfast for a midmorning snack. An early-morning exerciser, for instance, may want to have fruit or juice before he works out, followed later by something more substantial.

What foods you pick for a midmorning snack really depend on what works best for you, Dr. Wurtman says. If you're a carbohydrate craver, this is the time for a muffin, rice cakes, crackers, or a bagel without butter. If you know protein will restore you, try a hard-boiled egg, a piece of cheese, or a cup of yogurt.

If you're someone who prides himself on getting through the morning on sheer nerve, you might think breakfast is a bother, at best. But, nutritionists agree, even long-time breakfast skippers who start eating a morning meal begin to feel like they have the wind at their backs. Their morning becomes a breeze.

Protecting and Restoring Your Good Health

Old-Fashioned, Doctor-Approved Cold Remedies

The more scientists learn about the common cold, the more it appears that Grandma was right. Kaiser-Permanente, the nation's largest health-maintenance organization, consulted experts on colds and flu at several leading medical centers. Here is their advice for self-treatment.

Rest ● Grandma was right when she said, "Rest." The effort required to fight a cold, especially during the first few days, is the equivalent of hard physical labor, which is why colds cause lethargy. Take it easy. If possible, stay home for a day or two. In most cases, there's no need to get into bed, but rest helps spur self-healing. It also isolates cold sufferers, which limits transmission.

Bundle Up ● Another of Grandma's classic recommendations, bundling up helps alleviate the chills associated with fever.

If You Smoke, Stop ● Smoking irritates the inflamed naso-pharynx, depresses blood levels of vitamin C, and paralyzes the respiratory cilia, which move mucus out of the infected area. Impaired cilia mean that mucus falls into the lower respiratory tract, increasing the risk of complications.

Drink Eight Ounces of Hot Liquids Every Two Hours ● Hot fluids soothe an irritated throat, help relieve nasal congestion, and prevent dehydration. Don't drink cold beverages. One study shows that they impede the movement of nasal mucus and contribute to congestion.

For Sore Throat, Gargle with Warm Saltwater, Suck on Hard Candies and Increase Relative Humidity ● The recommended salt mixture is ½ teaspoon per eight ounces. Any hard candies may help, but if you'd like extra pain relief, look for lozenges that contain the FDA-approved anesthetics discussed in "OTC Sore-Throat Relief." Humidify your immediate surroundings with a hot bath or shower, by inhaling steam, or with a vapor-izer or humidifier. Consult a physician if swallowing becomes a problem or if you have a sore throat and a fever over 101°F with no other cold symptoms; this might be strep throat.

For Fever, Headaches, and Body Aches, Try a Cool Cloth on the Forehead or use Acetaminophen or Ibuprofen ● Be sure to drink plenty of fluids. Seek professional help for fevers above 101°F, fevers above 100° that last more than two days, or any fever with rash, stiff neck, severe headache, and/or marked irritability or confusion—this might be meningitis, a poten-tially fatal condition of the fluid surrounding the brain and spinal column.

For Nasal Congestion, Drink Hot Fluids, or Try a Vaporizer, Hot Bath or Shower. At Night Use Extra Pillows to Elevate the Head ● If you must take something, use a single-action de-congestant, unless you're pregnant or nursing or have high blood pressure, heart disease, or a history of stroke, in which case consult your physician.

OTC SORE-THROAT RELIEF

Packaged as lozenges, gargles, or sprays, over-the-counter sore-throat remedies provide temporary relief from minor pain. They do not kill cold viruses or speed healing. The sore-throat remedies approved by the Food and Drug Administration are not recommended for more than two days of continuous use. If pain persists or becomes more severe, consult a physician.

Several anesthetics have proved safe and effective for cold-related sore throat.

- Benzocaine.
- Dyclonine hydrochloride.
- Salicyl alcohol.
- Benzyl alcohol.
- Hexylresorcinol.
- Phenol (sodium phenolate).

In lozenges, these drugs typically begin to work within 1 to 5 minutes and provide relief for 10 to 30 minutes. They may be taken every two hours. Aspirin, which relieves inflammation, may also help.

For Runny Nose, Use Disposable Tissues ● Cold viruses cannot survive long in paper tissues. But cloth handkerchiefs harbor live virus and recontaminate the fingers with virus each time they are used. Wash your hands after blowing your nose or after wiping a child's nose. If you must take something and you're convinced that antihistamines help you, take a single-action product—preferably one with a low risk of drowsiness. (If you're pregnant or nursing, you should consult your physician.)

Do Not Suppress Productive Coughs. For Dry Coughs, Use a Vaporizer, Take Hot Showers, Suck on Hard Candies or Get an OTC Remedy with Dextromethorphan ● Consult a physician if a productive cough brings up brown or bloody sputum, if a dry cough lasts more than two weeks, or if any cough is accompanied by fever, chills, chest pain, wheezing, or short-ness of breath. These symptoms might indicate pneumonia.

Avoid Timed-Release Medications ● Timed-release pills may seem more convenient, but studies show that the reality falls short of the promise. The medication is not released uniformly. You may get too much for a while, then too little. It's better to take shorter-acting drugs more frequently.

Nature's Prescriptions for Your Heart

Recent headlines have sizzled with the hot news about heart disease and aspirin. They were sparked by a study reported in the *New England Journal of Medicine* showing that 11,037 doctors who swallowed a buffered aspirin tablet every other day for five years suffered only half as many first heart attacks as doctors who didn't take aspirin. Thus, this drug lurking in every medicine chest was hailed as a new proven deterrent to the nation's number-one killer.

Behind the good news, though, some heart experts made every effort to ensure that a few important points didn't get lost. Point one: Aspirin therapy isn't for everyone; check with your doctor if you think you might benefit from such a preven-tive program. Point two: The study examined the protective effect of taking one aspirin every *other* day; taking aspirin more frequently doesn't necessarily translate into more pro-tection—it could be less. And point three (perhaps the most important of all): Don't let the news about aspirin overshadow the importance of other nondrug, natural methods of heading off heart trouble—methods that are increasingly prescribed by cardiologists and family physicians. And because of new re-search, these heart helpers have been making a few headlines of their own.

Here's the latest news on nine of them.

Fiber-Pack Your Diet

A recent study has confirmed what scientists have suspected for years: People who eat the most dietary fiber (in foods like whole grains, fruits, and vegetables) have the lowest death rates due to heart disease.

Scientists from the School of Medicine at the University of California, San Diego, gathered the confirming data by monitoring for 12 years the development of heart disease in 859 men and women over age 50. They discovered that the people who ate at least 16 grams of fiber a day had only one-third the risk of dying of heart disease as those who ate less than 16 grams. To put that into perspective: One-third cup of oat bran contains about 8 grams of fiber; two slices of whole-wheat bread, about 3 grams; and one-half cup of cooked corn, about 4 grams.

A surprising finding: People who were getting 18 grams of fiber per day had a 25 percent lower risk of dying of heart disease than those getting just 6 grams less.

Why does fiber seem to be protective against heart disease? Scientists are still looking for the answer. "We know that certain kinds of fiber, such as oat bran, are more effective in lowering cholesterol than other kinds," says Elizabeth Barrett-Connor, M.D., one of the study's investigators. "But we think that fiber does more for the heart than just lower cholesterol. It's been suggested, for example, that fiber might hinder the formation of blood clots that can lodge in the arteries causing heart attacks and strokes."

Begin an Easy-Does-It Workout Program

The old news is that regular exercise reduces your risk of heart disease. The new news is that you don't have to work yourself into the ground to get this benefit. So say recent studies that document the good-for-your-heart power of moderate exercise, such as walking, bicycling, stair climbing, and slow jogging.

A study of 5,930 men and women, for example, showed that those who regularly did easy-does-it exercise like walking and stair climbing had more healthy-heart factors going for them than the sedentary people. In general, moderate exercisers were less overweight or had lower blood pressure or had lower cholesterol and triglyceride levels than their less-active peers (*Preventive Medicine*).

And in the world of moderate-but-mighty workouts, walking has emerged as a new favorite. Maybe it's because news got around that a brisk walk is nearly as good for your cardiovascular system as a jog. Or because experts have been saying that walking just a few minutes a day, three or more days per week, is enough to do your heart a lot of good.

Bruce Gladden, Ph.D., of the University of Louisville's Exercise Physiology Laboratory, is one of those experts. He recommends walking for at least 15 minutes three to five days a week.

"You don't have to rely on speed alone to give yourself a good workout," he says. "Just look for a course with lots of grades and hills. Or try picking up the pace for 1 minute or so, and then go back to your regular pace. Just concentrate on finishing a 15-minute workout comfortably. If you're too out of breath to talk to your partner while you walk, you're probably going too fast. Conversation should be a little difficult, not impossible."

Get a Doctor's Prescription for Niacin

More and more doctors are prescribing the B vitamin niacin to their patients with heart disease. Why? Because study after study has confirmed niacin's ability to lower blood cholesterol and triglycerides. In fact, it's now standard therapy for people with genetically caused superhigh cholesterol. Some recent research highlights:

● In a study of over 8,300 men who had had heart attacks, 11 percent fewer deaths occurred among those who took niacin compared to those who did not. The data suggest that taking niacin may add 1.6 years to the lives of heart attack survivors.
● Another study of 101 heart patients revealed that the 62 who took at least one gram (1,000 milligrams) of niacin per day for an average of 11 months had significant improvements in their blood cholesterol values. Total cholesterol dropped an aver-

age of 18 percent, and high-density lipoprotein (HDL) cholesterol (the beneficial kind) shot up an average of 32 percent. People who took more than 100 milligrams but less than 1,000 milligrams experienced similar—but less dramatic— changes. Some researchers think that such manipulations of cholesterol may translate into fewer heart attacks and longer life.

● A research trial involving 162 men with heart disease yielded historic results. A significant number of those who were treated with a combination of niacin, a cholesterol-lowering drug, and low-fat diets actually experienced a *halt or reversal* in the progression of their disease.

"Niacin, or nicotinic acid, is becoming one of the drugs of choice for people who can't achieve satisfactory cholesterol reduction through a low-cholesterol diet," says Thomas Pickering, M.D., of the Helmsley Cardiovascular Center at New York Hospital.

He and a lot of other experts point out, however, that you should never take niacin in doses far above the U.S. Recommended Daily Allowance (20 milligrams) without medical supervision. In high doses, niacin is considered a drug and may have many druglike side effects—flushing, itching, stomach upset, changes in liver function, elevated glucose levels, and others. Your doctor may be able to minimize these. (By the way, niacinamide, a popular form of niacin, doesn't cause flushing—but doesn't affect blood fats either.)

Be Nice

For years, research suggested that Type-A people— competitive, hard-driving, achievement-oriented, irritable—are at risk for heart disease. But recent studies drew conflicting conclusions. So researchers looked further to try to identify some specific aspect of the Type-A personality, not the whole gamut of behaviors, that hurts the heart. Their investigations paid off. A new-evidence review by experts from the National Institutes of Health and others shows that research may have isolated the so-called toxic component of Type-A behavior.

It's hostility. People who are merely ambitious or driven aren't the ones at risk for heart disease, the data suggest. It's people who are hostile (not merely irritable)—rude, abrasive, cynical, vengeful, manipulative, or condescending toward others.

So if hostility is the real heartbreaker, the question is: Can a hostile person change from a hawk to a dove in time to prevent a heart attack?

It isn't easy. But Meyer Friedman, M.D., the "grandfather" of Type-A research, has been successfully helping Type A's get rid of their classic behaviors, including what he calls "free-floating hostility." His theory: To become less hostile you have to act less hostile.

Here are some of his tips for rooting out hostility.

● First, dump your personal myths about hostility—myths that you need hostility to get ahead in the world, that you can't change your hostile ways, that giving and receiving love is a sign of weakness.

● At least twice a day say to someone, "Maybe I'm wrong," whether or not you think you're in error.

● Go out of your way to express your affection and admiration for family members and make a point of accepting any tenderness they show you. Regularly buy a thoughtfully chosen gift for one of them.

● Make a conscious effort to employ understanding and forgiveness when you encounter people you don't like.

● Take time out every day to examine and appreciate something beautiful.

Drop a Little Weight

Scientists are bringing us both bad news and glad tidings about being overweight. Bad: Extra poundage is harder on your heart than expected. Glad: Dropping weight (even a little!) does more good than anyone realized.

"Being overweight is a more important risk factor in heart disease than we thought at first," says Joseph Stokes, M.D., of the Boston University Medical Center and the Framingham Heart Study. "It's a causative factor, partly because it raises blood pressure and cholesterol, which are risk factors in themselves."

But a new landmark Harvard University study of 1,400

overweight people reveals that those who lost just 10 percent of their body weight showed big decreases in symptoms of obesity-related diseases, including hypertension.

That confirms what many doctors have been finding out on their own. "We know that if one of our patients loses five pounds, chances are his blood pressure will be lower," Dr. Stokes points out. "A 1 percent reduction in body weight usually produces a two-point reduction in blood pressure, and that's a substantial change."

Develop a Preference for Fish

The effect of fish oil on heart disease is currently undergoing a scientific reassessment. Scientists are reevaluating whether adding fish oil to the diet can really help in the war against cholesterol. Some studies say yes, absolutely; others say maybe not. But on one thing most researchers do agree: Fish itself is heart food, for at least two reasons:

First, fish is lower in saturated fat (the enemy of the cardiovascular system) than beef, pork, or lamb—and thus is a good substitute for them. "There's no question," says Stuart Rich, M.D., a University of Illinois cardiologist, "eating fish instead of meat will lead to less coronary disease."

Second, the oils in many fish—oils containing large amounts of omega-3 fatty acids—are known to lower blood triglycerides, a blood fat linked to heart disease, especially in women.

So, the prescription from experts is to dine on fish at least twice a week.

Balance Your Sodium/Potassium Intake

You already know that some people can lower their high blood pressure by consuming less sodium. And you've probably heard that consuming more potassium may help hypertension. Now there's new research confirming that doing both is more effective than doing either alone.

In a study of over 1,300 men and women over age 30, researchers found that those who had a good "sodium/potassium ratio"—a balance of low sodium intake and high potassium intake—had lower blood pressures. The lower the ratio (that is, the lower the sodium intake in relation to potassium intake), the lower the blood pressure. And the lower the pressure, the lower the risk of stroke.

"As people consume more potassium, they excrete more sodium," says Dr. Barrett-Connor, a coinvestigator in the study. "This helps keep blood pressure down. But as people age, their kidneys become less efficient at eliminating sodium. Which means that shifting from a high-sodium to a high-potassium diet becomes more important."

Some top sources of potassium are potatoes, avocados, orange juice, raisins, sweet potatoes, tomatoes, squash, bananas, dried apricots, skim milk, sardines, flounder, and salmon.

Defat Your Diet

After decades of heart research, cholesterol is still public enemy number one. Dietary strategies often center around cutting out cholesterol-ridden foods. That's important. But what many fail to realize is that cutting our intake of saturated fat is even more critical. The fact is, saturated fat can drive up your blood cholesterol levels faster and higher than consuming cholesterol itself.

"Studies have shown that watching your saturated-fat intake is definitely more important than even cutting your cholesterol intake," says Dr. Pickering. "So you've got to be careful about those advertisements that say a product is 'cholesterol-free.' What they're not telling you is the more crucial factor—how much saturated fat there is."

All this puts a different light on food selection. Foods once considered taboo—shellfish, for instance, because of their high cholesterol content—may actually be less harmful to the arteries than foods like chocolate or hydrogenated vegetable shortenings, which are low in cholesterol but high in saturated fats.

Get to the Source of Your Stress

Most people probably figure that someone under heavy stress is begging for heart trouble. And they may be right, researchers say. Stress has been linked to heart attacks and "sudden cardiac death." And there's evidence that stress may actually boost your cholesterol levels and throw your blood fats out of balance.

So stress busting is heart smart. The standard antistress prescriptions include exercise, relaxation techniques, meditation, and breathing exercises—methods for defusing your reactions to stress. But experts have also been issuing new recommendations aimed at snuffing out whatever causes stress in the first place. Here's some of their advice.

● Don't assume that life in the fast lane is necessarily stressful. Doctors from Harvard Medical School, authors of *Your Good Health,* say that calling a hectic pace stressful may actually cause stress where there is none. Research, they say, suggests that some busy people who work long hours may have less stress than less harried people trapped in dead-end situations. For some, the fast pace may be the best pace.

● Stop worrying about things that don't matter. Pinpoint what's really important and let the rest take care of itself.

● Rearrange your routine or environment. Sometimes simple changes in your schedule, workload, or surroundings can eliminate big sources of stress.

● Set realistic goals. Shooting for pie in the sky can lead to a sense of helplessness and hopelessness.

● Don't try to be perfect. You'll only set yourself up for failure—and, in the process, set yourself on a course of higher stress, even burnout.

Don't Let Your Lawn Make You Green at the Gills

Saturday afternoon you attacked crabgrass and grubs with the full force of modern chemistry. Another victory in the greening of America. But a few days later, your kid's wheezing, your dog's scratching at an oozing sore, you've got something that looks like athlete's foot, and here comes your neighbor clutching what you recognize as the dead remains of the forsythia bush he's been nurturing for five years.

The smoking gun is that spray can you used to apply weed and bug killer to your grass, the one that's dripping leftover pesticide onto your garage floor.

"The weekend gardener, with his handy, hand-pressurized, extinguisher-type canister sprayer with adjustable nozzle or his garden-hose attachment device, is a menace to the neighborhood." That's the unqualified opinion of D. J. Ecobichon, Ph.D., professor at McGill University in Quebec and pesticide expert. Dr. Ecobichon says that carelessly applied weed and insect sprays—known jointly as pesticides—have been known to cause eczema-like reactions, asthma attacks in people who don't have asthma, and property damage. They are also suspected of causing cancer.

"Nobody ever said pesticides were safe," points out Dr. Ecobichon. "By their very nature, all pesticides have some inherent degree of toxicity. They have to be toxic or we wouldn't be using them." Most insecticides, for instance, work on the bugs' nervous systems, and most insects' nervous systems are not that different from those of the higher animals, including man. So most insecticides will work on our nervous systems, too.

What worries Dr. Ecobichon most is the tremendous growth in the use of herbicides, or weedkillers. "Chemical companies will very gleefully tell you herbicides attack parts of plants with no counterpart in human beings," he says. "That's true, but many weedkillers are contaminated with toxic chemicals that form during the manufacturing process." One little slip of the temperature-controlling device and a company's herbicide brew starts cooking up things like dioxin, a potent environmental toxicant found in Love Canal and other waste dump sites.

Smart Spraying

But with proper care and intelligent shopping, you can avoid most of the potential health hazards. Dr. Ecobichon recommends these precautions:

Measure Chemicals Carefully ● Follow the directions on the label when mixing pesticide concentrate with water. Too much pesticide will burn your lawn and is more dangerous to handle. Be especially careful when you open the container not to splash the concentrate, which is more than ten times as toxic as the mix, according to Dr. Ecobichon.

Cover Up ● When you mix up a batch of pesticide, wear gloves, a rubberized apron or coveralls, boots and a full-face shield. Goggles don't cover enough. "It only requires 30 seconds of stupidity to spend many years in pain," says Dr. Ecobichon. "A little splash of diluted pesticide will give you a rash, but a little splash of concentrate could take your skin off." Better yet, if you have only a small area to spray, use a premixed solution.

Keep a Source of Running Water Nearby ● Wash spilled pesticide off skin, clothes, and boots promptly, and dilute any pesticide spilled on the ground. Emulsifiers and solvents in the concentrate can be as harmful as the active ingredient and will actually cause the pesticide to be absorbed faster through your skin.

Wear Shoes When You Spray ● Rubber shoes are the best, but they may be hot to wear. Heavy leather is okay as long as you're not going to stand in the sprayed grass too long. "People routinely spray in their sandals, then wonder why their feet break out," says Dr. Ecobichon. "The rash looks like athlete's foot."

Be a Good Neighbor ● Let people living nearby know what you're going to spray and when. "You could be a nice guy and send their kids off for ice cream," suggests Dr. Ecobichon. And if a neighbor has a chemical sensitivity, wait until he's out shopping or away from home for the weekend and spray then.

Don't Spray on Windy Days ● Aerial drift from sprayed-on pesticide has been known to turn friendly neighbors into the Hatfields and McCoys. Pesticides meant for lawns can be fatal to surrounding shrubbery, so wait for a calmer day.

Evacuate Kids and Pets ● And don't forget Fido's food and water dishes. "I've seen dogs and cats who have lain down on sprayed lawns get rashes on their bellies," says Dr. Ecobichon. "They start scratching and then you've got a bigger problem." How soon is your lawn safe for children and other living beings? Dr. Ecobichon says water-soluble solids that can be kicked up stay on the grass for about three days. After that, they become fixed to the grass blades and aren't a problem. You can speed up the "fixing" process by watering your lawn thoroughly 24 hours after you spray.

Don't Eat or Smoke ● Hands are the easiest ways to get pesticide into your mouth. Once you've started, don't take a lunch break until you're done.

Clean It Up ● Wash your hands and clothes when you're done, and clean out your spray can before you store it. Rinse empty pesticide containers, then break glass ones, and puncture metal and plastic containers so they can't be used again. Empty bags and cardboard boxes should be torn up and thrown away. Trying to burn empty pesticide containers can be a big mistake. "If you are downwind of the fire, you could inhale volatile vapors," warns Dr. Ecobichon. "I saw a case of malathion toxicity happen that way—a seriously poisoned man who got smoke full in the face."

Build Bones to Last a Lifetime

You lift a perfect pot roast out of the oven; bend to tie a child's shoelace; pull ripe carrots from your garden. Simple, everyday tasks—for most of us.

But for people with osteoporosis, these same enjoyable activities can fracture a bone.

A fall, blow, or lifting action that would not normally bruise or strain the average person can easily break one or more bones in someone with severe osteoporosis. The condition affects 15 to 20 million individuals in the United States. As many as half of all American women over 45 years of age and 90 percent of women over 75 have osteoporosis to some extent. This bone-thinning disease is the reason behind some familiar "signs" of aging that often begin in the fifties or sixties—a gradual loss of height, an aching and curved back, or hips or wrists that break easily.

Osteoporosis is a "silent" disease because it develops with no symptoms before these signs occur. What's more, the condition is difficult for doctors to diagnose early—before it causes problems.

There is good news, however: It is possible that osteoporosis and the fractures it causes can be prevented or at least delayed. Scientific evidence has suggested some measures women can take—with the support of their doctors—that may prevent or at least slow down the development of osteoporosis. These measures can be adopted whether a woman is in her thirties, fifties, or seventies. They can be helpful for men at risk for osteoporosis as well.

Those at Greatest Risk

A number of risk factors for osteoporosis have been identified.

Being a Woman ● Osteoporosis—as evidenced by vertebral fractures—is estimated to be six to eight times more common in women than in men. To begin with, women develop less adult peak bone mass than do men. For several years after menopause, women also lose bone much more rapidly than men do, due to a fall in their bodies' production of estrogen.

Early Menopause ● This is one of the strong predictors for the development of osteoporosis, especially if menopause is induced by surgery or other means that remove both ovaries or cause a sufficient drop in estrogen. Many experts define "early" menopause as menopause occurring before the age of 45.

Being Caucasian ● White women are at higher risk than black women, and white men are at higher risk than black men. Some experts estimate that by age 65 a quarter of all white women have had one or more fractures related to osteo-porosis. Oriental women are also thought to be at greater risk for the disease, but there are not enough data to confirm this.

A Chronically Low Calcium Intake ● Because calcium is so important to building and maintaining bones, inadequate intake can put you at risk.

Lack of Physical Activity ● However, exercising at an extreme level that halts menstruation in a young woman also may lead to bone loss.

Being Underweight ● While this is a risk factor in this instance, it is *not* meant to suggest that being overweight is a good idea. Both overweight and underweight people are better off trying to attain their desirable weight.

Other *possible* risk factors include:

● A family history of osteoporosis.
● Smoking cigarettes.
● Excessive use of alcohol. It is not known exactly how much alcohol is too much, in terms of osteoporosis, but alcoholics may be at risk for the disease.

Causes of Osteoporosis

Living bone contains a protein framework (the osteoid matrix) in which calcium salts are deposited. In fact, the bones and teeth contain about 99 percent of the calcium in the body. Calcium makes bone hard.

Bone, like many other tissues of the body, is constantly being rebuilt or "remodeled." Old bone is torn down, "resorbed," and replaced with new bone in much the same way that people remodel buildings by tearing out and replacing walls.

This process of bone resorption and remodeling serves two purposes: It keeps the skeleton well tuned for its mechanical uses, and it helps to maintain the body's balance of certain essential minerals such as calcium. The body keeps a relatively constant level of calcium in the blood, because important biological activities such as contraction of muscles, beating of the heart and clotting of blood require quite constant blood levels of calcium.

When the blood calcium level drops, more calcium is taken out of bones to maintain the appropriate level. When the blood calcium level returns to normal, increased amounts of calcium are no longer taken from the bones.

As a person grows during youth, bones are metabolically active, and calcium is deposited into bone faster than it is taken out. The deposition of calcium into bone peaks at about 35 years of age in men and women. At the time of "peak bone mass," the bones are most dense and strong.

Some experts believe that the level of bone mass at this age may help determine whether a person may later lose enough bone to fracture easily. If a young woman achieves a high peak bone mass—possibly through increased calcium intake, moderate weight-bearing exercise, and other lifestyle choices—she may be less likely to develop osteoporosis later. But we need much more information on this important point.

During a person's late thirties, after peak bone mass is attained, bone loss begins and the bones become less dense. This occurs naturally and gradually in both men and women. In addition, as women and men age, their bodies generally begin to absorb less calcium from food.

Given the complex factors that influence bone, there may be many ways in which osteoporosis can develop. Current data point to two strong contributing factors: a drop in estrogen levels in women due to menopause (technically known as "estrogen deficiency") and a chronically low intake of calcium ("calcium deficiency"). The scientific evidence is stronger for estrogen deficiency than for calcium deficiency.

Menopause ● As a woman passes through menopause, her body's production of sex hormones declines and menstruation gradually diminishes until it stops altogether. (If menopause occurs because of removal of the ovaries, the drop in estrogen is relatively sudden.) Hormones are chemical substances produced by glands to control organ activities. Estrogen, the female hormone, seems especially to influence bone substance by slowing or halting bone loss. It may also improve the absorption of dietary calcium by the intestine.

This role of estrogen makes biological sense. During the childbearing years, a woman needs a strong skeleton and a healthy reserve of calcium in case she becomes pregnant and later nurses children. After menopause, she no longer has the same need for this protective reserve of calcium. As her estrogen level drops, her bones start to contribute a larger share of calcium to meet the body's needs.

Too Little Calcium in the Diet ● Some scientists believe that a chronic shortage of dietary calcium is one important factor leading to osteoporosis. Each day, adults lose some calcium in the urine and feces and, to a lesser extent, through their skin. If these losses are not balanced by adequate amounts of calcium in the diet, "the body goes to the 'bank,' " as one expert put it, "and the bank, of course, is the skeleton." The bones begin to break down to maintain the proper blood level of calcium.

Other Causes ● Certain diseases or drugs can lead to bone loss. A doctor can evaluate a person who has one of these disorders or is taking one of these drugs, and work with her to avoid osteoporosis. These include:

● Medications such as corticosteroids (to treat arthritis and other diseases) and heparin (an anticoagulant).
● Diseases such as hyperthyroidism, hyperparathyroidism, kidney disease, and certain forms of cancer (lymphoma, leukemia, and multiple myeloma).
● Impaired ability to absorb calcium from the intestine, caused by diseases of the small intestine, liver, or pancreas.
● Excessive excretion of calcium in the urine.

Symptoms

In most cases, a patient is 50 to 70 years of age when osteoporosis is diagnosed. The disorder, however, can strike a woman as early as in her midthirties.

Crush fractures of the vertebrae can occur with or with-

out causing pain. Thus, other clues to the presence of osteoporosis besides back pain are loss of height or curvature of the
upper back. However, a chronic aching along the spine or,
more often, pain from spasm in the muscles of the back may
occur. With a partially collapsed spine, the muscles of the
back must take a greater share of supporting the upper half of
the body, so these muscles may "complain."

Prevention and Treatment

In recent years, scientists have identified several measures that may help reduce the toll of osteoporosis. The measures discussed here were described in the 1984 National Institutes of Health Consensus Development Conference on Osteoporosis.

It should be noted that estrogen replacement is the only
one of these measures in which there is well-documented
evidence of effectiveness in the prevention of fractures from
osteoporosis. Although complete proof is lacking that the
other measures—such as increased calcium intake—prevent
bone loss leading to fractures, many believe that current data
are sufficient to suggest that these measures be adopted.

Many of these measures can be taken throughout life
to promote healthy bones. (Exceptions include estrogen-
replacement therapy for postmenopausal women.) It is possible that young women could build a high peak bone mass to
reduce the risk of developing osteoporosis. Middle-aged and
older women may be able to keep osteoporosis from occurring
or progressing. Men too may lessen their risk of osteoporosis.

Note: All of these measures are best undertaken with the
advice of a doctor.

Estrogen-Replacement Therapy ● For women at risk of osteoporosis, a doctor may prescribe estrogen when the body's
production of the hormone drops during and after menopause.
Menopause occurs naturally around the age of 50, although it
can occur when a woman is in her late thirties or into her early
sixties. Menopause will also occur if the ovaries are removed
by surgery.

Many experts feel that, in terms of its effects on osteoporosis, the benefits of estrogen replacement outweigh its risks. The decision to use estrogen, however, is one that should be made carefully by a woman and her doctor.

On the side of benefits, there is good evidence that low-dose oral estrogen is highly effective for the prevention of osteoporosis in women. Estrogen reduces the amount of bone destruction and thus slows or halts postmenopausal bone loss. It cannot, however, restore bone mass to premenopausal levels. Studies have shown that women who have begun taking estrogen within a few years after the onset of menopause have fewer hip or wrist fractures and possibly fewer spinal fractures than women who do not take estrogen. Even when started as late as six years after menopause, estrogen therapy reduces further loss of bone.

There is also scientific evidence that estrogen-replacement therapy confers some protection against cardiovascular disease. It is thought to raise blood levels of HDL (high-density lipoprotein) cholesterol and to lower LDL (low-density lipoprotein) cholesterol. Raised HDL levels and lowered LDL levels are associated with lower rates of heart and blood vessel disease.

On the risk side of the ledger, estrogen-replacement therapy is thought to increase the risk of a type of uterine cancer known as endometrial cancer from 1 per 1,000 women to about 4 per 1,000 women. Endometrial cancer, fortunately, is relatively easy to detect and treat, and it is rarely fatal. It is not a problem for a woman who has had her uterus removed, of course. Estrogen is not linked to breast cancer, according to most studies. The therapy may also increase the risk of blood clot formation (thrombosis).

There is little information on the *long-term* risks or benefits of estrogen combined with progestin in postmenopausal women. Studies on *younger women* taking progestins in birth control pills have shown an increased risk of high blood pressure and of disorders of the heart and blood vessels. Moreover, some progestins may blunt or do away with estrogen's protective effects against heart disease.

Until more data on the risks and benefits of estrogen replacement are available, doctors and patients may prefer to reserve estrogen (whether or not it is combined with a progestin), for situations in which there is a moderate to high risk of osteoporosis.

Premature menopause—especially through surgical removal of the ovaries several years before the time of natural menopause—places a woman at high risk of osteoporosis. Postmenopausal women having the risk factors mentioned earlier other than an early menopause may also want to discuss estrogen therapy with their doctors.

The recommendations above apply mainly to Caucasian women. Women of other races and their doctors might consider estrogen on a case-by-case basis. There is no good evidence that elderly women should be started on estrogen therapy to prevent osteoporosis.

Increased Calcium Intake ● An intake of calcium of 1,000 milligrams per day—through diet or diet plus supplements—might be beneficial in helping to protect against development of osteoporosis.

People, particularly women, should get plenty of calcium in their diets throughout life. Certainly children and teenagers need an adequate calcium intake as they and their bones are growing.

Studies show that the usual intake of calcium for adult women (ages 25 to 74) in the United States is 450 to 550 milligrams per day. This is well below the current Recommended Dietary Allowance (RDA) of 800 milligrams per day for women and men who are over 18 years old. Furthermore, studies cited by the 1984 NIH Consensus Development Conference on Osteoporosis led the conference panel to offer the opinion that the RDA for calcium is too low, especially for postmenopausal women, and may well be too low for elderly men.

The panel recommended that women consume the following amounts of calcium each day.

● Premenopausal and older women receiving estrogen need about 1,000 milligrams of calcium per day for calcium balance, that is, to keep the amount of calcium in the bones constant.

● Postmenopausal women (that is, all women past the age of menopause) who are not on estrogen need about 1,000 to 1,500 milligrams of calcium per day.

In addition, men who increase their calcium intake may prevent age-related bone loss as well.

In essence, with the exception of pregnant and nursing women, it is recommended that adult women and probably men should have a total daily intake of 1,000 milligrams of calcium, and women who are past menopause and not on estrogen therapy, may need up to 1,500 milligrams daily.

If the average American woman consumes an estimated 500 milligrams of calcium per day based on her current eating habits, then an additional 500 to 1,000 milligrams are needed; that is roughly the amount of calcium in two to four servings of milk or several servings of other calcium-rich foods.

It can be helpful to consult a doctor, registered dietitian, or nutritionist, who can estimate the amount of calcium in your usual diet. Then he or she can suggest ways to increase calcium in your diet and can recommend calcium supplements, if necessary, to bring the daily intake up to 1,000 milligrams.

A word about calcium-rich dairy products and dieting: The American diet is generally high in fat and efforts should be made to reduce fat intake. Consumption of low-fat dairy products reduces both fat and calories in the diet while supplying valuable calcium.

People who have difficulty digesting milk (as in lactase deficiency or lactose intolerance) might try eating yogurt or drinking milk that has been treated with the enzyme lactase (known as Lactaid) so it can be digested. Some yogurts contain lactase naturally.

For some people, it may be difficult to reach the daily levels of calcium intake suggested previously without taking calcium supplements. Different formulations of the supplements contain different amounts of elemental calcium, so it is important to read the product label. Calcium carbonate, for example, is 40 percent calcium. That is, 100 milligrams of calcium carbonate contains 40 milligrams of calcium, or "elemental calcium." In the case of calcium lactate (at 13 percent calcium), 250 milligrams of the compound would contain about 34 milligrams of calcium.

Calcium supplements are often in the form of tablets. Chewable tablets and powders may be available. One source of calcium carbonate is oyster shells, so this compound is sometimes called "oyster-shell calcium." Certain antacids contain calcium carbonate; in fact, one popular brand is virtually 100 percent calcium carbonate with only added sweeteners and flavorings. Other antacids with calcium carbonate also contain aluminum, which can hamper the intestine's ability to absorb calcium from food.

It is wise to consult a doctor to determine how much calcium you currently consume, whether you should take calcium supplements, and if so, what type. The number of calcium preparations on the market is growing steadily, and there is no one supplement that can be uniformly recommended. If you cannot get enough calcium in your diet and you must take supplements, here is some information to keep in mind.

● A recent study found that absorption of calcium from calcium carbonate is impaired in people with little or no stomach acid, which is common in people over 60. However, the scientists found that in these people absorption improved if the compound was taken with meals.

● Drink a full glass of water when taking a calcium supplement. (In general, it is a good idea to drink several glasses of water each day.) Levels of calcium intake greater than those recommended previously (1,000 to 1,500 milligrams per day) can cause kidney stones in susceptible people. Thus, people with a history of kidney stones should take calcium supplements only with a doctor's guidance. These people should be especially careful to drink plenty of water.

Normal Levels of Vitamin D ● Vitamin D is required for optimal absorption of calcium in the intestine. People who get very little sunlight exposure are at risk of vitamin D deficiency. This particularly applies to older people who may be confined to a home or nursing facility.

Scientists recommend 400 international units of vitamin

D each day. Most people get enough of this vitamin by being outside during the day and eating a normal diet. (Vitamin D is produced by the body naturally when a person is exposed to the sun.)

Fifteen minutes to an hour of midday sunshine may meet the daily need for this vitamin. Food sources include vitamin D-fortified milk, vitamin-fortified cereals, egg yolks, saltwater fish, and liver.

The phrase "normal levels" is important here. Taking *high* doses of vitamin D can have dangerous effects. No one needs to take more than the RDA per day without a doctor's guidance.

Moderate Weight-Bearing Exercise ● Send an astronaut into the weightlessness of space for an extended period of time and he or she will lose some bone mass. Likewise, lead a sedentary lifestyle and your bones will weaken in time from lack of force put on them.

"There's evidence that regular weight-bearing exercise can help increase your peak bone mass at maturity," says William Peck, M.D., physician-in-chief at the Jewish Hospital of Washington University in St. Louis, Missouri. "Also, exercise may help reduce the rate of bone loss in later years.

"Although exact amounts haven't been determined, your bones probably need at least an hour of exercise four times a week to benefit," Dr. Peck says. "Walking is an excellent, safe form of weight-bearing exercise." Some other good choices are tennis, hiking, race walking, jumping rope, aerobic dancing, racquetball, cross-country skiing, ballroom dancing and, to some extent, bicycling.

Keep in mind a few cautions about exercise. It's a good idea to consult a doctor before starting a program, especially if you've got heart, joint, or other problems or if you've been sedentary for a long time. Exercise programs should also be started slowly and built up gradually. Avoid excessively strenuous workouts that may damage bones.

Some young women who do an exceptional amount of exercise (such as vigorous long-distance running) may stop menstruating. If so, recent evidence indicates they may be at higher risk of osteoporosis.

Doctors encourage patients with osteoporosis to remain

as physically active as possible. It's important to avoid sudden strains from jumping or twisting, however, and situations where a fall might occur.

Prevention of Fractures

There are ways that people can make fractures less likely to occur, especially if their bones are already fragile. Minimizing hazards in the home can help, such as avoiding slippery floors and loose throw rugs, removing objects that might cause a fall, providing adequate lighting, and adding handles or nonslip bottoms to bathtubs. Railings on stairways inside and outside of the home can help.

It is also a good idea to avoid actions that stress the bones unduly. In particular, do not lift while bending forward. Lifting this way creates an unusual and unnecessary strain on the vertebral column.

A person should carry any weight close to the body, squatting and lifting straight up, using the legs and not the back. If the spine is weak, it is wise to completely avoid lifting heavy objects.

As has been described, recent research shows that fractures from having fragile bones may *not* be an inevitable part of life for postmenopausal women or older Americans. Studies are yielding new information about bone biology and are providing new methods of diagnosis and treatment if osteoporosis develops. In the meantime, there are steps that can be taken—beginning immediately—to protect the bones.

The Yeast Syndrome: Is It for Real?

For nine years, Lisa Waldbaum, a 33-year-old office worker, suffered heartburn, gas, constipation, painful joints, recurrent vaginal infections, fatigue, depression, upper respiratory infections, and skin rashes. She consulted numerous physicians, who prescribed antibiotics for her infections and steroids for her rashes, but nothing seemed to help.

When she was bothered by yet another vaginal infection,

she decided to try a new alternative women's health center rather than return to her regular gynecologist. The nurse-practitioner told Lisa she might be suffering from yeast syndrome, a chronic form of systemic yeast infection (candidiasis). The nurse referred Lisa to a physician, who confirmed the yeast diagnosis. He prescribed a diet low in yeast and sugar and oral nystatin to kill the yeast, and took her off steroids and birth control pills. After three months, Lisa's symptoms disappeared and she felt better than she had in years.

Did Lisa actually suffer from chronic yeast syndrome? Or did she simply have a variety of complaints that eventually resolved on their own? Most physicians dismiss yeast syndrome. But a growing number of M.D.'s—and many alternative practitioners—believe candidiasis has become a serious health concern.

Yeast Controversy

Candida albicans, the same microorganism that causes the "cottage cheese" type vaginal infections in women, is alleged to cause chronic yeast syndrome. *Candida* organisms are everywhere, and virtually everyone carries yeast in their intestinal tract. Yeast-syndrome proponents claim that diets rich in refined sugars and yeasted bread products, and heavy or prolonged use of antibiotics, steroids, and birth control pills cause an overgrowth of normal yeast and the destruction of other beneficial bacteria in the intestinal tract. They say yeast cells systemically invade the body, releasing a toxin that impairs the immune system and causes behavioral changes. Chronic yeast infection has been blamed for a wide variety of symptoms including acne, allergies, gastrointestinal complaints, skin rashes, fatigue, arthritis, premenstrual syndrome (PMS), depression, migraine headaches, and loss of libido. These and other complaints, say advocates, persist until the systemic yeast infection is treated.

Yeast syndrome first received national notice in the early 1980s with the publication of *The Missing Diagnosis* by C. Orian Truss, M.D. But it was pediatrician and allergist William G. Crook, M. D., author of *The Yeast Connection,* who sparked the almost evangelical zeal with which the alternative health movement has embraced yeast syndrome.

The alternative medical marketplace has been quick to respond. Numerous yeast syndrome clinics have sprung up around the country. Health food stores carry a variety of antiyeast products such as Cantrol, Yeast Fighters, Candida-Guard, and Candida Cleanse. Chronic yeast syndrome has become a hot media topic. *Redbook* magazine recently suggested that up to 10 percent of the population suffers from this new mystery ailment. Some proponents even claim that immuno-suppression from yeast overgrowth may explain why some infected with the HIV virus develop AIDS and others do not. They suggest that antiyeast therapy can help AIDS victims, many of whom are heavily overcolonized with yeast.

Widespread Problem?

Candida albicans exists in two forms: benign and budding (mycelial fungal form) that produces rootlike structures (rhizoids) which can penetrate mucous membranes. Rhizoid penetration of the intestinal tract allows other substances in the gut to invade intestinal tissues and causes widespread immune problems. Yeast overgrowth in the gut also blocks absorption of nutrients.

For reasons not entirely understood, *Candida* overgrowth is more common among women. One factor may be the use of birth control pills, which changes the vagina's pH and promotes yeast overgrowth.

Yeast-syndrome proponents claim that 30 percent of the population suffers from yeast-induced gastrointestinal and urinary tract problems, allergic/immune problems, emotional and mental difficulties, and hormone/endocrine difficulties. Pamela Morford, M.D., a Minneapolis gynecologist, says 90 percent of her PMS patients suffer systemic yeast infection.

Those who believe in yeast syndrome charge that orthodox medicine ignores the cause of many yeast-related problems and treats only the symptoms such as vaginal infections. Practitioners who embrace yeast syndrome attempt to stop yeast overgrowth by correcting the imbalances that caused it.

Orthodox medicine contends there is no evidence to support the yeast syndrome theory. For several decades, however, medical authorities have recognized the connection between certain health problems such as depression and the overgrowth of *Candida.* The so-called "drunken yeast syndrome," in which depression is caused by the internal production of alcohol by yeast, has been medically documented since the 1950s. Although yeast-syndrome critics concede that, because of the widespread use of antibiotics yeast overgrowth is more common now, they contend that *Candida* does not cause the broad range of symptoms proponents claim.

One of the strongest attacks on yeast syndrome has come from the American Academy of Allergy and Immunology (AAAI), which was quick to point out that the theory has not been tested with double-blind studies and that there is no published work to support either the theory or the antifungal treatment of yeast overgrowth. They warn that there are no effective diagnostic tests for yeast syndrome and that the overuse of antifungal agents causes side effects and may spur the growth of drug-resistant yeast strains.

A common complaint among critics of yeast syndrome is that proponents overdiagnose the problem. Even when the diagnosis is accurate, they contend, many practitioners fail to treat it properly. An article in the *New England Journal of Medicine* described the case of a two-year-old boy with candidiasis who was sent to Mexico for treatment with sheep-cell infusions and isoprinosine, a drug to boost the immune system. When the boy was finally treated with the antifungal agent ketoconozole, his throat and fingernail yeast infections quickly cleared up.

Despite their skepticism, even yeast critics concede that diet is connected to yeast overgrowth. Diabetics, for example, are at greater risk for chronic vaginal yeast infections because they have high sugar levels in their urine, which provides food for yeast growth.

Recently, some orthodox medical critics of yeast syndrome have softened their stand and have called for research into the syndrome. In a recent commentary in the *Journal of the American Medical Association*, Edward R. Blontz, Ph.D., of the University of Minnesota writes, "It must be determined if chronic candidiasis is widespread within the general population . . . It is imperative that well-designed studies are undertaken to unravel this mystery."

Skimpy Research

Research into chronic yeast is crucial if the syndrome is to ever be acknowledged by orthodox medicine. To date, there are no double-blind studies that support the theory or its treatment.

Much of the research cited by proponents comes from Kazuo Iwata, M.D., chairman of microbiology at Meija College of Pharmacy in Tokyo. Iwata, who has studied yeast since 1967, has isolated Canditoxin (CT) from yeast strains. CT injected into mice causes behavioral changes and immunosuppression.

Another much-cited expert is Steven S. Witkin, Ph.D., of Cornell University Medical School, who wrote an article in *Infections in Medicine* in which he claimed to have found immunosuppression and auto-antibody formation in patients with candidiasis. Witkin says he found headache, fatigue, bloating, and depression in patients with abnormal *Candida* antibody test results, and that they responded well to antifungal therapy.

Diagnosis and Treatment

Diagnosis of yeast syndrome is made, in part, from the individual's health history. *Yeast Connection* author Dr. Crook has developed a "Candida Questionnaire and Score Sheet" which asks questions about use of antibiotics, birth control pills and steroids, and symptoms such as vaginal infections, skin rashes, and emotional complaints. Although many yeast syndrome enthusiasts use the questionnaire, there are no reliable data to support it.

Laboratory diagnosis of candidiasis is even more controversial. Some experts say stool analysis is useless because most of the population has stool yeast. Others contend that blood tests aren't helpful because of the lack of standardized testing, the common occurrence of yeast antibodies among healthy people, and the lack of established *Candida*-specific antibody measurements.

One of the most accurate tests currently available is the IgA, IgM, and IgG *Candida* antibody test developed by Edward

A. Winder, M.D., of San Leandro, California. This test measures the levels of A antibodies, those secreted by mucous membranes; M antibodies, which are the first antibodies produced in response to foreign invaders; and G antibodies, long-term antibodies produced by B-cell lymphocytes. Other tests are being developed to detect immune complexes circulating in the bloodstream.

CandaScan, a new stool candidiasis detection test, claims to count the yeast in the stool and test its sensitivity to antifungal drugs. The test is too new, however, to be evaluated.

The goals of yeast-syndrome treatment are to kill the yeast and to correct the conditions that caused the initial overgrowth. The hallmark of yeast syndrome therapy is the anti-*Candida* diet coupled with an antifungal agent to kill the yeast. The diet calls for limiting the intake of yeast-based products and refined sugars. Dr. Crook suggests eliminating fruit for two weeks because of its high sugar content. John Trowbridge, M.D., coauthor of *The Yeast Syndrome,* recommends two weeks of the MEVY diet—meat, eggs, vegetables, and yogurt.

The most common yeast-killer is the prescription drug nystatin. It kills on contact by disrupting yeast cell membranes. It is relatively nontoxic and inexpensive ($5 per 100 tablets). It is usually prescribed in powdered form—½ teaspoon every six hours. Ketoconazole is the next most common antifungal agent. However, it is expensive ($40 to $70 per 100 tablets), potentially toxic to the liver, and dangerous for people with alcohol problems. Other prescription antiyeast agents include miconazole (Monistat), amphotericin (Fungizone), griseofulvin (Fulvicin), clotrimazole (lotrimin), and fluctosine (Ancobon). A few doctors are experimenting with Tricophyton-Candida-Epidermophyton (TCE) immunotherapy, a type of "allergy shot" for candidiasis.

Another yeast-treatment strategy involves using *Lactobacillus acidophilus* supplements to reseed the intestine with "good" bacteria and fight the yeast overgrowth. However, Keith Sehnert, M.D., who has treated more than 100 people for yeast-related problems, warns, "Not all *Lactobacillus* supplements are the same." He recommends the DDS-1 brand from

UAS laboratories. Dr. Sehnert says, "Most of the research on the health benefits of acidophilus have used DDS-1."

Since 1946, caprylic acid, a derivative of coconut oil, has also been used to treat yeast infections. Supplements of biotin and oleic acid, a fatty acid present in olive oil, appear to prevent the conversion of benign yeast into the invasive type. The recommended treatment is 300 micrograms of biotin with two teaspoons of olive oil three times a day. Garlic is another nutritional remedy touted for its antiyeast properties.

Herbs have also been used against yeast. Mathake tea, which uses a plant grown in the Fiji Islands, has been used with some success. A more popular herbal treatment is Taheebo tea, also known as Pau' D'Aroc of Lapacho, an ancient Inca remedy derived from the bark of South American trees. The active ingredient in Taheebo tea is lapachol, a quinine-acting drug used by the Chinese in antimalarial formulas.

A combination product called Yeast Fighter contains *Lactobacillus,* garlic extract, caprylic acid, and biotin in an herb tea blend. It is now available in health food stores.

Most people recover from yeast syndrome within ten days. Some, however, may take months or even years to improve. Some suffer from a relatively harmless flulike reaction within two to five days of starting treatment due to the massive destruction of yeast.

Other treatment recommendations include avoiding caus-ative factors such as antibiotics and steroids. Women who use birth control pills should switch to an alternate form of birth control or take *Lactobacillus* supplements to prevent yeast overgrowth. And male partners should be treated to prevent sexual transmission of yeast infections.

Is there anything to the yeast connection? It's a little premature to say for sure. Certainly proponents need to curb their claims that antiyeast treatment is a cure-all. And skeptics need to be open to the possibility that yeast syndrome is a 20th-century disease brought on by yeast-rich fast foods and our overdependence on birth control pills, antibiotics, and steroids. Only some well-designed research can answer the many questions this intriguing syndrome raises, but we must take it seriously.

Fact and Fiction
about Ulcers

An ulcer is a craterlike sore in the lining of the stomach, esophagus, or small intestine caused by excess stomach acid. How do you know if you've got one? The major symptom of an ulcer in the stomach is a burning, gnawing pain, usually felt throughout the upper part of the abdomen and sometimes in the lower chest. It usually occurs just after eating. The pain can last from half an hour to three hours and come and go, with weeks of intermittent pain alternating with short pain-free periods.

The more common form of peptic ulcer, the duodenal ulcer, is found in the first part of the small intestine, just below the stomach. It produces a gnawing pain that is usually confined to a small area in the upper-middle abdomen but sometimes radiates throughout the area. The pain is often temporarily relieved by eating but then returns one to two hours later and lasts for a couple of hours. It's often worse at night. Awakening with abdominal pain around 1:00 to 3:00 A.M. is a strong feature of a duodenal ulcer, although that can also indicate other problems, says Denis McCarthy, M.D., professor of medicine at the University of New Mexico in Albuquerque. You should see your doctor if you experience mild discomfort that lasts more than two or three days; it could mean a serious problem.

Setting the Record Straight

There are many common beliefs about ulcers, but not all of them are valid. Here are the facts.

Spicy Foods Irritate Ulcers, so You Should Stick with a Bland Diet ● This is false. Spicy or fried foods generally don't provoke ulcers unless you are particularly sensitive to them. And milk may actually aggravate ulcers because it stimulates acid production. Your best bet is to avoid the known acidic foods like coffee (even decaffeinated), tea, alcohol, and highly acidic fruit juices (like orange juice).

A High-Fiber Diet May Protect against Developing Ulcers ●
This is true. Studies have found that foods rich in fiber (such as
fruits, vegetables, and whole grain breads) not only protect
against developing ulcers but also promote healing and prevent relapses once ulcers do exist. It is believed that the fiber
somehow slows down or buffers the stomach acid.

How You Eat May Affect Ulcer Development ● This is true.
Eating slowly and chewing well mean less swallowed air, less
food intake, and less chance of irritating the stomach lining.
Three moderate-sized meals (no eating on the run or late at
night) reduce acidity in your stomach.

Ulcers Run in Families ● This is true. In fact, if your parents were prone to ulcers, you have a high risk of developing
one, too.

There is an Ulcer Personality ● This is controversial. Some
believe there may be one personality type that is uniquely
prone to ulcers. They think it's related to how people cope.
People who internalize their stress and anxiety tend to be more
prone to ulcers than those who let out their emotions on a regular and consistent basis.

   Whatever the case, it may be wise to learn ways to express
your feelings and to include a daily dose of stress management.
Progressive relaxation, exercise, deep breathing, massage, and
biofeedback all may lead you in the right direction.

**Crushed Aspirin Is Less Irritating to the Stomach Than Whole
Aspirin** ● This is false. If you are prone to ulcers, avoid
aspirin in all forms—even in cold remedies. Be aware that
other anti-inflammatory drugs and common menstrual medications may also aggravate the stomach lining, advises Janet
Elashoff, Ph.D., of the Center for Ulcer Research and Education in Los Angeles.

New Drugs Can Cure Ulcers ● This is false. There's a whole
spectrum of drugs with which your doctor can custom-tailor
your treatment, ranging from over-the-counter antacids to

prescriptions (like Tagamet) that suppress acid production. Most ulcers heal in 8 to 12 weeks if you take the medication as prescribed. Usually the side effects, such as diarrhea and drowsiness, are mild. But healing ulcers is not curing them, points out Dr. McCarthy.

Ulcers have a nasty habit of recurring. The best way to keep that from happening to you is to determine which foods cause you problems and to avoid them. Also learn to handle your stress.

Smoking May Cause Ulcers ● This is true. Smoking promotes ulcers of the duodenum—the section of the small intestine just below the stomach and the site of most ulcers—and delays their healing. Apparently, smoking inhibits the release of bicarbonate, a natural antacid, from the pancreas to the duodenum. Smoking may also cause the liquid parts of a meal to move out of the stomach and into the duodenum sooner than the solid parts of the same meal. Without the solid food to "buffer" the liquid food—that is, to neutralize its acidity—it is more likely to burn the duodenum and cause an ulcer.

Don't Catch Your Pet's Bugs

By Amy Marder, V.M.D.

Over the past decade, studies of the human/companion-animal bond have told us what many pet owners have always considered obvious: Pets are good for our health. Pets provide a source of constancy in our lives, give us companionship, make us laugh, and even exercise with us. All of these attributes enhance the quality of our lives and foster good health.

But pets occasionally do get diseases that sometimes are passed on to people. Should this be a cause for concern? For the most part, no. These diseases are rare, and there are many ways to prevent their transmission to people.

The greatest fear seems to have been generated by some claims that, fortunately, have very little evidence to back them up. A while back, for example, researchers found a statistical association between ownership of small dogs, the occurrence of canine distemper, and multiple sclerosis (MS). Subsequent studies have failed to duplicate those results. (Dogs should be immunized against distemper anyway, for their own welfare.) Also, because of the similarities between the AIDS virus and the feline leukemia virus (FeLV), some people have been concerned about catching AIDS from FeLV-infected cats. To date, there is no evidence to suggest that FeLV causes AIDS or any other disease in human beings.

Clamp Down on Bites

Animal bites are the most common pet-associated human health hazard in the United States. In a recent study the annual bite rate was estimated at 1 in every 170 people. Children are the most frequent victims, probably because of their unintentional bite-provoking behavior.

Most pet owners are well aware of the danger of contracting rabies from animal bites. Make sure that your pet's vaccinations are up to date.

Bites can be prevented through proper education, especially of children. Move slowly around animals and be gentle when petting and playing with them. Do not tamper with pets' food dishes and don't disturb them when they are sleeping. Don't approach stray animals. And when greeting an owned animal, always ask the owner if the dog is friendly before petting it. If a dog chases you, it's usually best not to run.

Good Pet Hygiene

There are several bacterial infections that can be passed from animals to their human companions. *Salmonella* and *campylobacter* are two examples. Both dogs and cats can harbor these bacteria even though they often show no symptoms. In people, though, infection can cause stomach upset and diarrhea. As with many gastrointestinal diseases, the key to prevention is proper hygiene.

Young children are most commonly affected, probably because of their less-than-sanitary habits. Children should be taught not to handle their pets' food or feces and to wash their hands after contact with animals, especially before eating (these bacteria are transmitted orally). That's good advice for adults, too. If your pet has diarrhea, separate the animal from your family and see your veterinarian.

Streptococcus, the bacterium that causes strep throat, is occasionally transmitted from a household dog. If a member of your family is having a problem with chronic strep throat, consider having your dog tested.

There are other bacterial diseases that pets can pass to humans, but they're much less common. Cat-scratch disease, or cat-scratch fever, is not serious and usually goes away without treatment. You can prevent it by avoiding cat scratches and bites and by not handling stray or unknown cats.

Leptospirosis, a disease that affects the kidneys and liver, can be passed on from dogs to people. The best method of prevention is annual vaccination of your dog so that he or she cannot become infected.

Yersinia pestis, the bacterium responsible for bubonic plague, is a problem in the southwestern United States. The disease is usually transmitted to man by fleas but can be spread directly from animals. Free-roaming pets are considered an important source of this disease, so keeping pets properly restricted is essential. Flea eradication also helps to prevent infection.

Some intestinal parasites of dogs and cats can be transmitted to humans, too, through feces. Roundworm (*toxocara*), hookworm (*ancylostoma*), and *Giardia lamblia* are examples. Again, for all intestinal parasites, good hygiene is key.

To prevent roundworm, a veterinarian should examine your pet's stool every six months for parasites. Most puppies and kittens are infected with roundworms at birth from their mothers and should begin treatment as soon as possible.

Another parasite, *Toxoplasma gondii,* is of concern to pregnant women because it can cause birth defects. People usually acquire the disease by eating raw or undercooked meat or by coming into contact with infected cat feces. Cats become infected by eating small rodents or birds.

Pregnant women should wash their hands thoroughly after handling cats, and should always wear gloves when gardening. Cat litter should be changed daily by a family member not at risk, and the litter box rinsed regularly in scalding water for five minutes. Pet cats should be fed adequate amounts of food and restricted from hunting, if possible. All meat should be cooked thoroughly, and hands, cutting boards, sinks, and utensils should be washed with soap and water after contact with raw meat.

Certain skin diseases can also be carried by pets. An extremely common one is ringworm, a fungal infection. Fleas, scabies, and other mites may also cause mild skin symptoms in people. All of these can be prevented by eliminating the infection on your pets.

Remember, simple preventive measures are usually all that are needed to protect yourself.

Heart Health Update: Prevention Is Paying Off

Quietly but steadily an exciting—and unexpected—health trend has gained momentum throughout North America. Twenty years ago, medical authorities would never have predicted it, but since 1968, the death rate from heart disease has plummeted 27 percent, saving an estimated 80,000 lives. That's a population larger than San Francisco's, or more than ten times the number of U.S. combat deaths in Vietnam. In 1968, the United States and Canada had the highest death rates from heart disease in the English-speaking world. Today, they have the lowest, and epidemiologists predict that many people alive today will live to see the day when heart disease is no longer North America's leading cause of death.

Everyone agrees that there are many reasons for the substantial drop in heart disease deaths. The question is, which factor is most important? Not surprisingly, a good deal of medical opinion divides along "party lines." Surgeons tend to credit the coronary bypass. Intensive care specialists favor coronary care units. Internists usually say a key factor has been increasingly aggressive drug treatment of hypertension and elevated serum cholesterol. Emergency medicine specialists laud improved paramedical response times and mass training in cardiopulmonary resuscitation (CPR). Public health officials favor the decline in smoking. Authorities in Type-A behavior point to stress management programs. Fitness buffs say it's aerobic exercise. And nutritionists credit lower-fat, lower-cholesterol diets. Every one of these factors plays some role, but recent studies agree that all the advances in high-tech medicine are nowhere near as important as simple, basic self-care. Lower-fat diet, exercise, quitting smoking, blood pressure control, and stress management have saved many more lives than bypasses, coronary care units, and the rest of modern medicine's high-tech wizardry.

Ischemic Episodes

"Heart disease" means atherosclerosis, the buildup of fatty deposits (plaques) on the walls of the coronary arteries, the blood vessels that nourish the heart. As atherosclerotic plaques develop, these arteries become narrowed (occluded), depriving the heart of necessary nourishment. Once coronary artery occlusion has progressed to a certain point, the malnourished heart suffers "ischemic episodes," periods when it receives too little food and oxygen to function properly. Chronic ischemia leads to the death of parts of the heart itself, and one or more of the four major types of heart disease: angina, myocardial infarction, cardiac arrhythmias, or congestive heart failure.

● Angina, also known as angina pectoris, is chest pain, a warning sign of impending heart attack. It may be mild or severe, and is usually associated with physical exertion.
● Myocardial infarction (MI or heart attack) occurs when a blood clot becomes lodged in an already-narrowed coronary artery, cutting off food and oxygen for an extended period, and causing portions of the heart to die. The classic heart attack causes crushing chest pain that radiates down the left arm and/or up under the jaw.
● Cardiac arrhythmias are electrical problems that disrupt the heart's beating sequence. A complicated electrical system triggers each of the heart's four chambers to beat. When this

electrical system malfunctions, the heart beats out of rhythm. Arrhythmias usually cause no unusual sensations, but occasionally the person notices heart palpitations or the feeling that the heart has skipped a beat. In healthy people, periodic minor arrhythmias are no cause for concern. But if heart disease has damaged the heart, life-threatening arrhythmias can occur.

● Congestive heart failure is heart exhaustion. The damaged heart becomes too fatigued to pump effectively, causing fluid accumulation in the lungs, labored breathing after minor exertion, and swelling of the feet and ankles.

Heart disease is insidious. For years, often decades, no symptoms signal the progression of atherosclerosis. Those who develop symptoms are the lucky ones. Angina, congestive heart failure, nonfatal myocardial infarctions, and detected arrhythmias can be treated. But most heart disease deaths occur suddenly and without warning. In about 500,000 cases a year, the first symptom is also the last. The medical term is sudden cardiac death, and the victim simply drops dead from a massive heart attack.

Surprising Figures

From 1920 through the 1960s, the death rate from heart disease rose dramatically. In 1968, heart disease caused 35 percent of U.S. deaths, but by 1982 the figure had dropped to 28 percent, and it continues to fall today. Equally impressive is the scope of this trend. Heart disease deaths are dropping in men and women of all ages and races.

Another way to track the decline in heart disease deaths is in rising life expectancy. Life expectancy remained stable throughout the 1960s, but it began to rise in the 1970s as deaths from heart disease started to fall. During the decade of the 1970s, North American women gained 2.5 years of life expectancy (to 78.1 years) and men gained 2.7 years (to 70.7). No other country has matched the United States/Canadian record against heart disease. In Germany, Scotland, the Soviet Union, and many other countries, heart disease deaths have not fallen at all; in quite a few they have increased. Apparently North Americans are doing something very right—but what?

The decrease in heart disease deaths caught the medical community by surprise. At first many researchers dismissed it as a statistical fluke. The news seemed too good to be true. It wasn't until 1978, ten years after the decline had first been documented, that the trend was officially recognized as real—but no one knew why.

At first glance, figuring out why does not seem particularly challenging. If heart disease incidence (number of new cases) decreases, then the falling death rate must result from preventive measures such as diet and lifestyle changes. If, however, incidence remains stable or increases, then the drop in deaths must be the result of improved medical technology.

Unfortunately, the situation is not that simple. No one knows the incidence of heart disease. It usually causes no symptoms until it's been present for many years. In addition, the downward trend in heart disease deaths has been deduced largely from analyses of death certificates, which are notoriously unreliable. The only way to pinpoint cause of death is by autopsy, and autopsy rates have been falling steadily for many years. When autopsies are performed, pathologists find that the cause of death as listed on the death certificate is often incorrect.

High-Tech Care

Since 1968, when the death rate began to fall, the treatment of heart disease has been revolutionized. Coronary care units (CCUs) are among the most important innovations. The first CCUs were developed in the early 1960s when cardiologists realized that heart attack sufferers who survived the first 12 hours had a good chance of recovering. CCUs are short-term intensive-care units that focus a tremendous amount of medical technology on the immediate aftermath of heart attack in hopes of keeping victims alive for those crucial first 12 hours. Once stabilized, heart attack survivors are then moved out of the CCU and treated less intensively. Studies show that CCUs have cut in-hospital heart disease death rates by 15 to 30 percent.

That looks very impressive, but it's actually less so. Many people who survive heart attacks thanks to CCUs still die from heart disease weeks, months, or years later, so it's difficult to count CCU discharges as lives "saved." In addition, as CCUs have proliferated—most hospitals now have them—an increasing proportion of patients hospitalized with coronary problems have been admitted to them, including those with mild heart attack, whose survival prognoses are better to begin with. But it's impossible to separate the lives truly "saved" by CCUs from those who would have survived without high-tech interventions. After taking these confounding factors into consideration, several studies have concluded that CCUs account for only about 13 percent of the decrease in heart disease deaths.

About 60 percent of heart disease deaths occur before the person reaches a hospital. In the last 20 years, paramedical programs that provide emergency life support out in the community have become increasingly sophisticated. A small army of paramedics has been deployed. Response times in some communities average less than five minutes. Thanks to the revolution in computer microelectronics, many paramedical vehicles are now equipped with machinery once available only in hospitals. And literally millions of people have been trained to administer CPR, which can keep heart attack victims alive until professional help arrives. But studies in Seattle, which boasts a very sophisticated paramedical program and an aggressive CPR training program, show that in a population of two million, such out-of-hospital intervention programs save only about 100 lives a year. Only a small proportion of the North American population is served by advanced life support paramedical teams. Authorities estimate that paramedical programs are responsible for no more than 4 percent of the decline in heart disease deaths.

Coronary bypass grafting was one of the major surgical innovations of the 1970s. A portion of artery from the leg is used to reroute blood around severely occluded portions of the coronary arteries. About 140,000 such operations are now performed annually at a cost of tens of millions of dollars a year. Bypass surgery relieves angina pain effectively, but it remains unclear to what extent it contributes to long-term survival. Most authorities estimate that it accounts for only about 5 percent of the drop in heart disease deaths.

Heart transplants and artificial hearts have received a

great deal of publicity. But these marvels are available to only a very small number of people after the heart has been so extensively damaged that there is no other alternative. Meanwhile, there are 750,000 heart disease deaths each year.

Prevention

The controllable risk factors for heart disease include high serum cholesterol, smoking, chronic high blood pressure (hypertension), obesity, sedentary lifestyle, and Type-A behavior.

North Americans have changed their eating habits significantly in the last decade. In a recent U.S. Department of Agriculture poll, half of those surveyed said they had changed their diet because of health concerns. From 1950 to 1980, per capita consumption of eggs (high in cholesterol) dropped more than 30 percent. Lard consumption fell 80 percent and butter 55 percent. High-fat red meats and whole milk are also down; lower-fat chicken, fish, and skim milk are up. These dietary changes have reduced the average U.S. cholesterol level by more than 7 percent since 1960. This may not sound like much, but studies estimate that the decrease in serum cholesterol may account for as much as 30 percent of the decrease in heart disease deaths.

The public health campaign against smoking has been gaining momentum since the Surgeon General's 1964 report that urged the nation to quit. In the 1950s, about half of Americans smoked. Now less than a third do. Smokers who quit begin to reduce their risk of death from heart disease almost immediately. The decline in smoking is responsible for about 24 percent of the decline in heart disease deaths.

Treatment of hypertension became a public health priority in 1973 when the National High Blood Pressure Education Program was launched. Before then, hypertension was largely undetected, untreated, and uncontrolled. Now department stores sell blood-pressure cuffs for self-monitoring at home. And the dangers of high blood pressure have been widely publicized. Low-fat diet, moderate exercise, stress management, and a variety of drugs can reduce high blood pressure. Regular exercise and stress management to control Type-A behavior (hostile, competitive, always time pressured) also contribute to hypertension control. About half of those with hypertension are diagnosed, treated, and under control. There's still room for improvement, of course, but authorities estimate that the control of hypertension has reduced heart disease deaths about 8.5 percent.

While scientists generally agree about these figures, the data supporting them are purely epidemiological, which leaves some room for doubt. If one could demonstrate a falling *incidence* of heart disease in addition to the falling death rate, the case for prevention through diet and lifestyle changes would become compelling. Recently a 25-year study of 6,285 DuPont employees has shown just that. In the group that made significant lifestyle changes, heart attacks, both fatal and non-fatal, dropped 28 percent. A similar study of subscribers to the Kaiser-Permanente health-maintenance organization in California showed a drop in heart attack hospitalizations of 27 percent. Finally, a New Orleans study shows that from 1964 to 1972, the period when the country in general made heart-sparing lifestyle changes, autopsies there turned up a corresponding decrease in atherosclerosis.

The Bottom Line

In this era of skyrocketing medical costs and finite health resources, it's important to look at the financial aspects of the decline in heart disease deaths. Medical interventions are effective only after preventive efforts have failed. Prevention costs much less per person, and it's for everyone, while high-tech medical advances help a smaller and smaller proportion of the population as self-care becomes our way of life. CCUs, bypasses, and artifical hearts may keep some people with heart disease alive longer, but they do nothing about underlying heart disease. Risk-factor reductions, however, mean that the heart stays healthy and does not require as much medical intervention, if any. Like the old saying goes, "If it ain't broke, you don't have to fix it."

Examining the estimated contributions of the various factors that contribute to the decline in heart disease deaths, the figures reveal that medical interventions appear to account for 32 percent, with lifestyle changes accounting for 62.5 percent, and 5.5 percent unaccounted for.

Risk-factor reduction isn't as flashy as, say, the artificial heart. But it works a lot better. No doubt *Time* and *Newsweek* will continue to miss the point and focus on "amazing medical breakthroughs." But take heart. Throughout North America, people are getting the real message. Prevention is the way to go.

CREDIT WHERE CREDIT IS DUE

Here is a summary of the contributions of various factors to the decline of heart disease deaths.

High-Tech Factors	
Coronary Care Units	13.0%
Paramedics and CPR	4.0%
Bypass Surgery	5.0%
Medical Treatments	10.0%
Heart Transplants	negligible
Artificial Hearts	negligible
Subtotal	**32.0%**
Lifestyle Factors	
Blood Pressure Control	8.5%
Quit Smoking	24.0%
Lower Cholesterol	30.0%
Subtotal	**62.5%**
Unknown	5.5%

---

21 Ways to Tame Warm-Weather Allergies

When crocus and other spring flowers have arisen, so have allergenic molds, pollinating plants, allergy-inducing insects and a few other allergy triggers you wouldn't suspect in a million years.

But not to worry. There are effective ways to deal with these little buggers so you can celebrate fun in the sun with a dry nose and itchless eyes. Here are 21 antiallergy strategies from the experts.

1. Know what you're dealing with. Determine whether your sneezes and sniffles result from an allergy attack or a seasonal cold or flu. Colds and flu, explains the American College of Allergists, come with a fever, sore throat, thick nasal discharge, aches, and chills. Antihistamines, prime antiallergy medicine, won't help these ills.

True allergies generally involve lots of sneezes (often in rapid succession); a thin, watery nasal discharge; itchy eyes, nose, or throat; postnasal drip; ears that pop or feel plugged; loss of smell and sinus headache. Antihistamines often do help.

The final clue to the difference is that a cold or flu rarely lingers longer than a week. Allergy attacks don't end until the source (such as pets or pollen) is gone.

2. Keep cool, not cold. Experts warn that setting an air conditioner on "superfreeze" may aggravate allergy symptoms. Better to set the temperature switch at a comfortable 70°F.

3. Shortcut lawn maintenance. Cut grass pollen by cutting the grass. Botanist James Thompson, Ph.D., of Miles, Inc., explains that "it's the bloom that releases allergy-aggravating pollen spores. And most lawn grasses can't bloom if they're kept clipped." Two exceptions are annual bluegrass and Bermuda grass. "They'll bloom even with a crewcut," says Dr. Thompson.

"In most cases, however, just keep the grass trimmed to three inches and minimize watering; you'll keep pollen levels low." Luckily, pollination isn't necessary for a healthy lawn.

4. Become a masked mower. If you mow the lawn yourself, wear a mouth-and-nose mask. Mowing can kick up a lot of pollen and molds. Masks like the kind that home renovators wear to keep from breathing dust are perfect. (Painter's masks, though, may have openings that are too big to stop pollen.) They're available at many hardware stores and home centers for under $3.

"Make sure it fits tightly," says Dr. Thompson. "And don't be tempted to reuse it. The inside may become contaminated with pollen the instant you take it off."

5. Groom vacant lots. An average vacant lot can produce almost 22 pounds of pollen in less than a week. These lots are especially hard on allergic children who play outdoors, says Dr. Thompson.

If you have such a lot in your neighborhood, call city hall, find out who owns the land and insist that they keep it mowed. (Many areas have laws requiring such mowing.) If that fails, appoint yourself caretaker. The rewards may be substantial. Many allergists feel that people sensitive to pollen suffer more when such fields are nearby.

6. Avoid pollen's peak times. Pollen levels are always low after a rain. Otherwise, the safest time for outdoor activities depends on where you live, say researchers from the United Kingdom.

Rural pollen counts generally peak around 3:00 P.M.—when the temperature is high, the sun is shining, the wind is strong, and the humidity is low. In the city, pollen counts peak a good four hours later. It seems that all the heat generated by buildings and people keeps the pollen aloft until the cool of the evening allows it to settle to the streets below.

7. Watch those rings and things. Nickel allergies are fairly common, especially, it seems, in the spring and summer months. British researchers found that the amount of nickel released from jewelry, metal buttons, clasps and the like is greatly increased by perspiration. So, if you're allergic to nickel, don't be surprised to find your symptoms worsen as the weather warms up. And, if you've never suffered from a nickel allergy before, don't be surprised if you do now. To lessen your risk, keep the metal as cool as possible, limit the time the nickel's in contact with your skin and use an alkaline barrier cream underneath jewelry.

8. Shower. The most effective first-aid treatment for a pollen overdose is already in place in your home. It's a shower.

"Medications aren't going to help much if your hair and clothes are still covered with pollen," explains Dr. Thompson. "But a quick shower that rinses away the pollen will often minimize the reaction. It's even better if you can soak down with a hose while you're still outside. That way, you won't bring any airborne pollen into the house."

9. Shampoo. "When you're outdoors, your hair acts like a giant filter, capturing and holding lots of windblown pollen," Dr. Thompson adds. "That's why it's important to wash your hair as soon as you come in from working outdoors." This is especially true if you've been mowing the lawn. "Your hair can actually pick up a static charge during mowing," explains Dr. Thompson, "and cause more pollen to attach itself and cling tight."

10. Decontaminate your auto air conditioner. Everyone with pollen allergies knows to close the car windows and turn on the air conditioner when the air is heavy with pollen. Unfortunately, many car air conditioners are heavily contaminated with mold.

Most of the mold is emitted in a short burst when an air conditioner is first turned on. You can avoid the problem by running the air conditioner for a while with the vent closed and the car windows open—preferably without you in the car. Or, for a more convenient solution, decontaminate your air conditioner. You can get the service at most GM and Ford service centers for around $75.

11. Pretreat for protection. Even allergic asthmatics can garden, says Richard Farr, M.D., former allergist for the National Asthma Center. Using your inhaler *before* you go out not only prevents an immediate reaction but may have long-term benefits as well. One of Dr. Farr's patients pretreated himself faithfully for several years, and now his outdoor asthma is gone.

Some allergic people without asthma may use the same tactic, says Lyndon Mansfield, M.D., of the Texas Tech Health Science Center. He explains that taking an antihistamine before heading outside may prevent an allergy attack.

12. Stop poison ivy with a garden hose. About 85 percent of us are allergic to poison ivy, oak, and sumac. Thank goodness, the antidote is usually close at hand: water.

"If you think you've been exposed on a picnic or a hike, take a dip in a stream or soak yourself with a hose," says dermatologist William Epstein, M.D. "If you act fast enough, you'll have no reaction."

If you do come down with that telltale red, blistery rash, Dr. Epstein strongly suggests that you wash everything that you may have touched while contaminated with the plant's allergenic oil. "One patient of mine kept getting poison ivy over and over again for weeks," says Dr. Epstein, "until he realized it was all over the steering wheel of his car."

13. Dry up your dust mites. The warm, moist air of springtime triggers a population explosion in dust mites, the biggest cause of indoor allergy problems. Dust mites live deep inside your furniture and rugs. Housecleaning *can't* get rid of them, but dry air can.

Richard Weber, M.D., chief of the allergy/immunology division at Fitzsimmons Army Medical Center, explains that mite populations drop off dramatically in winter when the air in the house is dry. In spring and summer, use dehumidifiers and air conditioners to keep these pests under control.

14. Fashion a hypoallergenic wardrobe. Many modern fabrics (such as permanent press) are treated with formaldehyde to keep them wrinkle-free. But the combination of warm days and high humidity can release that formaldehyde. The result may be an itchy contact-allergy rash. So, look for fabrics that are formaldehyde-free—like 100 percent synthetics, silk, linen, or fabrics that have been mercerized, sized, or Sanforized.

15. Try shift work. People who take a beating from outdoor allergens should plan to do their outside work in several short shifts of around 15 minutes each, advises Dorothea Linley, M.D., a gardener for more than three decades. "If you try to do it all at once, you'll get tired and start breathing heavily," she explains. "And heavy breathing increases the rate at which you're inhaling allergens."

16. Stay clear of things that sting. If you're allergic to insect stings, you have to try harder than most to avoid them. The biggest springtime stingers, explains entomologist Miles Guralnick, are paper wasps. "They're irritable when they're nest building," he says. Honeybees begin zipping around as soon as the temperature hits 57°F. Later in the season, yellowjackets make piles of firewood and wood chips risky places.

Whatever the flying felon, "freezing in place" is the *worst* thing to do when attacked, says Guralnick. Instead, exploit the beast's poor eyesight and dodge between buildings or trees.

17. Head off a bad reaction. If you have had a serious reaction to an insect sting (hives, difficulty breathing, shock), it means that the next sting might be your last. Immunotherapy (allergy shots) around 16 times a year conveys almost total protection. Yet David Golden, M.D., of Johns Hopkins University, says that 90 percent of the people who know they're at risk *don't* get the shots, which explains why 50 people die from allergic reactions to stings each year. Don't be one of them. If you've had a bad reaction, ask your allergist about the shots *and* carry an emergency kit.

18. Check your sunscreen. People with sensitive skin might want to avoid sunscreens that contain PABA. It's a well-known cause of contact-allergy reactions. To complicate matters, if you develop a PABA allergy, you may also find yourself allergic to the topical anesthetic benzocaine as a result. The reverse is true, too. Using benzocaine topically, especially on damaged skin, can trigger an allergy to benzocaine and to PABA.

19. Beat the itchy-mouth syndrome. Food allergies sometimes relate to pollen allergies. Swedish researchers explain, for example, that many people with birch-pollen allergy experience an itchy sensation in their mouths after eating apples, carrots, hazelnuts, peanuts, cherries, peaches, plums, potatoes, and walnuts. Likewise, some people who are allergic to mugwort react to celery, melons (especially watermelon), and apple. Ragweed-allergy sufferers may be sensitive to melons and bananas. And those with grass-pollen allergies sometimes find melons, oranges, peas, and tomatoes difficult to swallow.

Luckily, say the researchers, allergy shots that control the pollen problems also control the oral itching. In addition, they note that allergic reactions occur with *fresh* foods only. Most people with the allergy can eat the same foods safely if they're cooked or canned.

20. Don't show off your shorts (or sheets). Taking advantage of a little springtime sunshine to dry the wash is a great way to bring the fresh scent of outdoors inside. Unfortunately, it can bring airborne pollen in, too. Clothes dryers avoid this outdoor contamination.

21. Don't go topless. A California physician actually tested a hardtop (with windows up and air conditioning on) versus a convertible (with top down) for pollen invasion. During a leisurely drive through the wine country, 3 pollen grains reached the hardtop's passenger seat; 143 hit the same spot in the convertible.

Sun Sense, Skin-Wise

There was a time when soft, porcelain-white skin, protected forever from the sun, was considered a sign of great beauty and affluence.

There was a time when skin cancer was not an epidemic.

It's no coincidence. Research has proved that sun exposure is the major cause of the wrinkled, mottled skin once blamed only on aging—and, worse, that overexposure is responsible for 90 percent of the most common forms of skin cancer.

The good news is that you have the power to save your own skin. With a little foresight (and a few simple precautions), you can enjoy seasons in the sun without suffering damaging effects.

There's good news too for the unfortunate people—over half a million of them—who do get skin cancer each year. With early detection and treatment, all types of skin cancer are curable. Looking ahead, there's even an experimental vaccine on the horizon. To learn more about the bright future for your skin, read on.

Three of a Kind

The most common and curable skin cancers—basal-cell and squamous-cell carcinomas—are caused by overexposure to the sun's ultraviolet rays, specifically the ones called UV-B. These same rays that toast your skin to a golden-brown color can disrupt the vital genetic material (DNA) in your skin cells, causing cancer. And, if you double your exposure to UV-B, your risk actually triples or quadruples. Apparently, skin that's already damaged may be more vulnerable to additional doses of UV-B.

Fortunately, basal-cell and squamous-cell carcinomas tend to be slow growing and rarely spread to other parts of the body. Still, left unchecked they can cause severe tissue damage and should not be taken lightly.

The most dangerous form of skin cancer is called malignant melanoma. It can be life-threatening if not detected in its early stage. There's some pretty convincing evidence to suggest that melanoma is also related to sun exposure. First, melanomas appear to be more prevalent the closer you get to the equator, where the sun is strongest. "The melanoma rate in Arizona is three times the rate in Boston," says Arthur Sober, M.D., associate chief of dermatology at Massachusetts General Hospital and a member of the medical council of the Skin Cancer Foundation.

Also, melanoma occurs more frequently on the legs in women and on the chest and back in men—areas more often exposed to the sun.

Interestingly, too, Dr. Sober's research points to an association between severe sunburn and melanoma. People who had blistering sunburns as adolescents were twice as likely to develop the disease as people who never got burned. This suggests that brief, intense sun exposure holds more melanoma risk than the long-term, occupational exposure of farmers or sailors, for example.

From Sun Wary to Sun Worship

The population of the United States increased 10.6 percent between 1980 and 1987. The number of new melanomas increased 83 percent during that same period, according to recent estimates by Darrell S. Rigel, M.D., of the New York University School of Medicine (*Journal of the American Academy of Dermatology*). Why the surge?

Around the middle of this century, the tables turned on tanning. Suddenly, bronze skin became a badge of wealth—a sign that you had the money and time to frolic in the sun. Sun worshipers of the 1960s and 1970s may be realizing the detrimental effects only now, says Dr. Rigel, since there is probably a lag period between ultraviolet damage to the skin and the appearance of melanoma.

Many scientists are convinced that the depletion of the earth's protective atmosphere (the ozone layer) will further increase future rates of skin cancer. The sun is getting stronger, in effect, because less of the dangerous rays are filtered out before they reach us.

Put Up a Sunscreen

Don't worry, though: You don't have to spend the rest of your life indoors. Though that would keep you out of harm's way, it's not conducive to an active, healthful lifestyle. So, rather than curtail your activities, consider these simple precautions.

● Shift your schedule. Stay out of the sun during the most dangerous period of the day. UV-B rays are strongest between 10:00 A.M. and 2:00 P.M. (11:00 A.M. and 3:00 P.M. daylight saving time) in most parts of the United States. So try to plan outdoor activities for the early morning or late afternoon.

● Wear protective clothing. Remember, if your clothes are sheer enough to see through, the sun can shine through, too. Long-sleeved shirts and long pants made of lightweight but tightly woven fabrics are best. And, always wear a hat, preferably one with a wide brim.

● Don quality shades. Skin cancer can occur on the eyelids, and several studies have linked cataracts to sun exposure. Other reports show that too much light exposure can also be harmful to the retina. So look for sunglasses that block at least 95 percent of ultraviolet rays, and 75 percent of visible and infrared light. (If the pertinent information isn't available on the tag or frame, ask the salesperson or call the manufacturer.)

● Use a sunscreen, rain or shine. Choose one with an SPF (sun protection factor) of at least 15 and apply it liberally every day. That's right, *every day!* Studies have shown that sun damage is cumulative. Every minute you spend in the sun—pulling weeds in the garden, supervising the kids at the playground, driving with your arm propped out the window—contributes to your chance of developing cancer. Also, the sun reflects off many surfaces, such as sand and concrete. So, even if you're shaded by an umbrella or hat, be sure to use a sunscreen on all exposed skin, including the backs of the hands, the tops of your feet, behind your knees, under your chin, on and behind your ears. And beware of overcast days: The sun's rays are just as damaging when it's dreary as when it's sunny. As much as 85 percent of ultraviolet rays can penetrate clouds. Apply sunscreen at least 15 minutes before going outside, to give your skin a chance to absorb it. Reapply sunscreen at least every two hours and after swimming or perspiring heavily.

● Protect your lips with an SPF-15 lip balm or block. Your lips can receive considerable sun exposure, but they have no protective pigment whatsoever. Long exposure to the sun can crack and discolor them, causing sores or blisters. And lips are a prime site for skin cancer.

● Don't hit the tan accelerator. There are some products that claim they can speed up the tanning process, reducing the amount of sun exposure it takes to build up a golden glow. According to some dermatologists, they simply don't work and are still being investigated. (Don't confuse tan accelerators with self-tanning lotions, which react with amino acids in the skin to create a safe tan without any sun.)

High-Power Protection

With the recent boom in the availability of ultrahigh-SPF sunscreens, you might be wondering if you should be looking to a higher power. After all, if SPF 15 is good, SPF 30 must be better, right? Yes, but only marginally better.

Unprotected, the average person's skin turns red after ½ hour of sun exposure. With proper use of an SPF-15 sunscreen, the average person can stay out 15 times that long, or 7½ hours, with the same effect (although that's not recommended), says Perry Robins, M.D., president of the Skin Cancer Foundation. "Since the sun is at its most dangerous for only about 4 hours, an SPF-15 sunscreen already leaves a wide margin of safety."

Never Too Late—Or Too Early

Since sun damage is cumulative, you might think that it's useless for an older person to practice prevention. Presumably, the damage is already done. Not so, says Dr. Sober. It's never too late. "You can't undo the damage that's done. But if you start protecting yourself at age 50 or 60, you can prevent additional damage from occurring."

It's never too early for sun protection, either. "People receive 80 percent of their lifetime sun exposure before the age of 20," says Dr. Sober. In a statistical study at Harvard University, Robert S. Stern, M.D., and colleagues concluded that regular use of an SPF-15 sunscreen during the first 18 years of life would reduce a person's risk of developing the most common skin cancers by 78 percent. "People should be protected from the sun from birth," says Dr. Sober. "Babies should be protected with a hat and umbrella until six months of age. After that, sunscreens should also be used."

All of this skin pampering can pay off double in the future. Not only can you cut your chances of developing skin cancer, but you can help preserve your skin's natural youth and beauty. While a tan may look good on you now, prolonged sun exposure produces the kind of damage that eventually makes skin look old. Blood vessels become more prominent, the skin yellows and becomes mottled. Damage to skin fibers causes loss of elasticity, leaving skin stiff and dry as leather, and setting the stage for wrinkles.

Are You a Sensitive Person?

Certain commonly used medications can make you overly sensitive to sun damage. In fact, many antibiotics, antide-pressants, diuretics, and other drugs can cause you to get an intense sunburn after only brief sun exposure. Ask your doctor or pharmacist whether any medications you may be taking could cause such a reaction.

Of course, some people's skin is naturally more suscepti-ble to sun-induced damage than others. Do you have blue, green, or gray eyes, blond or red hair, a light complexion or freckles? Do you sunburn easily or tan poorly? Have you had bursts of intense sun exposure? If you answered yes to any of those questions, you're at a higher risk for developing skin cancer and should be especially careful about protecting yourself.

Has a member of your family been diagnosed with melanoma? Then your chance of developing it is greatly increased. "Ten percent of people with a melanoma have another family member that is affected," says Dr. Sober. "The familial association is striking." Doctors know that the tendency to develop melanoma is transmitted genetically. The key here is that only the *tendency* is transmitted. So protection from the sun and early detection can really make a difference.

Some of the people who've inherited the tendency to develop melanoma don't know it, because they show no outward signs. But many people do. They have what's called dysplastic nevi—that just means unusual moles. The moles are generally larger than ordinary moles (greater than 5 millimeters in diameter, about the size of a pencil eraser), have irregular outlines, and uneven pigmentation or color. People who have these moles should be examined by a dermatologist, as should their family members, says Dr. Sober.

Another risk factor is a high number of moles. One study showed that a person with 11 to 25 moles has a 60 percent greater chance of being diagnosed with melanoma than a person with fewer than 10. The chance is 340 percent greater for people with 26 to 50 moles, and soars to 880 percent greater in people with more than 100 moles. Again, those people need to be especially careful to limit sun exposure and examine their skin frequently for signs of melanoma.

Take a Good Look at Yourself

At least 90 percent of all skin cancers detected are readily curable. The trick is to spot them early. So examine your skin regularly. Once a year is sufficient for most people. Do it on your birthday; then you won't forget. (People at high risk should examine their skin more frequently.) Make sure you don't miss any nooks or crannies. Use a hand mirror and a full-length mirror to check out hard-to-see places. Be alert to the following warning signs.

● A skin growth that increases in size—and appears pearly, translucent, tan, brown, black, or multicolored.
● A mole that changes color or texture, increases in size or thickness, or has an irregular outline.

● A spot or growth that continues to itch, hurt, crust, scab, erode, or bleed.

● An open sore or wound that does not heal, persists for more than four weeks, or heals and reopens.

If you notice anything the least bit suspicious, have it checked immediately by a physician, preferably a dermatologist or other skin specialist. "There is no reason to panic," says Dr. Robins. "But it is important to have it checked within a couple of days."

The most common treatment for skin cancer is surgery, and one technique in particular has generated quite a bit of excitement, according to Dr. Robins. It's called the Mohs technique, after its inventor, Frederic E. Mohs, M.D. There's been a recent explosion in its use for eradicating skin cancer. "About 100,000 people are treated this way every year," says Dr. Robins. "That's because it has a higher cure rate than any other treatment."

Mohs surgery (also known as microscopically controlled surgery) is done using a local anesthetic. The surgeon cuts thin layers of the malignant tissue and checks each layer under a microscope for the presence of tumor. The procedure is repeated until the tissue is tumor-free. "That way the cancer is traced to its roots, and the smallest possible amount of healthy tissue is sacrificed," says Dr. Robins. "The technique is used most for cancers located on the nose, eyes, or ears."

Other types of surgery, as well as radiation therapy, are also valuable in treating skin cancer. The kind of treatment used depends on the type, size and location of the cancer, as well as the patient's health.

A Fired-Up Defense

A lot of the research into the treatment and prevention of melanoma has focused on getting the immune system to fight back from within. One of the most promising prospects is a vaccine. "It's still in the developmental stages," says Jean-Claude Bystryn, M.D., professor of dermatology at New York University School of Medicine and director of the melanoma program at the NYU Kaplan Cancer Center. "This is the outcome of studies conducted about ten years ago where we showed that we could prevent melanoma in mice by immunizing them with a vaccine."

Several years ago, with funding from the Skin Cancer Foundation, Dr. Bystryn developed a similar vaccine for human melanoma. It's made from extracts of melanoma cells. "We've been conducting studies with people for the past few years," he says. "We've shown that the vaccine is safe and that it augments immunity to melanoma in about half of the patients we treat. But it is still too early to tell if we are having a favorable effect on the progression of the disease."

Melanoma arises in the skin cells that produce the pigment melanin, the one responsible for tanning. In a recent study, Dr. Bystryn and colleagues studied melanoma patients who had white areas on their skin—areas where pigmented cells had been destroyed. Those patients had a better chance of recovery from the disease, the doctors found (*Archives of Dermatology*). That's promising news for the development of a vaccine. "If the body has the ability to destroy a pigmented cell that is normal, it may have the same ability if that cell becomes malignant," says Dr. Bystryn, a member of the Skin Cancer Foundation Medical Council. "We suspect that this is the result of an immune process. If we can stimulate an immune response through vaccines, then maybe we can slow the course of melanoma or prevent it."

The Skin Cancer Foundation supports research and promotes public and medical education to help curb skin cancer. For more information and a free copy of the Foundation's newsletter, "Sun and Skin News," write to Skin Cancer Foundation, Box 561, Dept. S, New York, NY 10156. Please include a stamped business-size, self-addressed envelope.

Score Your Cholesterol Savvy

Why is it that when the subject of cholesterol comes up, half of us become so suddenly tongue-tied? Here's a topic that should be near and dear to our hearts—literally—but we can never remember which foods are high in cholesterol and which aren't. We know that cholesterol helps cause heart attacks, and we know that heart attacks await all too many of us. But, very often, we don't understand the subject well enough to save our own skins.

Some Timely Questions

Well, here is a chance to test and perhaps expend your knowledge of cholesterol. Below are ten multiple-choice and four true-or-false questions. Write down your answers, score yourself at the end, and find out how to prevent the heart attacks that remain out there in the future, lurking like sharks.

1. What exactly is cholesterol? (*a*) a mushy yellow substance found in the brains, liver, kidneys, and adrenal glands of animals, as well as in eggs; (*b*) a type of fat that is essential to the formation of cell walls within the body and necessary raw material for the production of sex hormones; (*c*) a food constituent that you could easily do without, since your body can synthesize all the cholesterol it needs from other sources; (*d*) all of the above.

2. Your blood work shows that you have a cholesterol level of 220. What should your response to that information be? (*a*) relief; (*b*) concern; (*c*) alarm.

3. True or false: A Porterhouse steak, served rare, is your favorite food, but you don't have to worry much about cholesterol because you run two miles a day, keep your weight down, and threw away your last pack of cigarettes several years ago.

4. What does the acronym HDL stand for, and what do HDL's do? (*a*) heavy-deuterium leukocytes; they seek and destroy cholesterol molecules; (*b*) high-density lipoproteins; they scavenge for cholesterol and help flush it out of the body; (*c*) hydrogen di-lymphocytes; they prevent cholesterol from being absorbed through the intestinal walls.

5. True or false: You've been eating the classic, high-fat western diet for 40 years, so it's too late for you to worry about high cholesterol. You might as well go on enjoying your favorite foods.

6. Some doctors believe that we should consume no more than about 100 milligrams of cholesterol each day. How much cholesterol does the average American currently consume per day? (*a*) 250 to 350 milligrams; (*b*) 400 to 500 milligrams; (*c*) 650 to 1,000 milligrams.

7. When you eliminate fats from your diet, such as red meat and peanut butter, are you eliminating cholesterol at the same time? (*a*) yes; (*b*) no; (*c*) sometimes.

8. True or false: Diet and lack of exercise can promote heart disease, but most people who develop this condition have an inherited predisposition to it. As one person put it, "The best way to beat heart disease is to pick the right grandparents."

9. The most immediate step you can take to lower the amount of cholesterol in your diet is to stop eating (*a*) Miracle Whip, tuna, egg whites, corn-oil margarine, olive oil, cottage cheese; (*b*) liver, red meat, butter, egg yolks, mayonnaise, ice cream, and coconut oil; (*c*) potatoes, beans, white-flour pasta, cookies, and other sweet baked goods; (*d*) all of the above.

10. On a business trip, you find yourself in a hotel restaurant. Before you've had a chance to recover from the plane ride, limo ride, and elevator ride, the waiter is asking you to choose the dressing you'd like on your tossed salad. Which of the following contains the least fat and cholesterol? (*a*) Roquefort/blue cheese; (*b*) Thousand Island; (*c*) ranch, with buttermilk and mayonnaise.

11. How much cholesterol does one egg yolk contain? (*a*) 125 milligrams; (*b*) 240 milligrams; (*c*) 320 milligrams; (*d*) none, since all of the egg's cholesterol is in the white.

12. True or false: Many people have had coronary bypass surgery and they emerged from it "like new." So you don't have to watch your cholesterol intake because if heart disease strikes, you'll have a bypass. That will take care of the problem.

13. It is not unusual for a man with a cholesterol count of 250 who smokes a pack of cigarettes a day and has high blood pressure to have a heart attack by the age of (*a*) 40; (*b*) 50; (*c*) 60.

14. How often should you have your cholesterol count measured by a doctor? (*a*) once a year, in the course of a complete physical exam; (*b*) once very two years; (*c*) very intermittently; if you are healthy, slim, and have no history of heart disease, frequent checks are not necessary.

Answers

Now check your answers with ours and find out how cholesterol-savvy you really are!

1. (*d*). On the one hand, cholesterol is a necessary building block for certain important tissues. On the other hand, a cholesterol-free diet would do us no harm at all. Eliminating cholesterol-rich animal foods would reduce our risk of heart disease without reducing our bodies' ability to form new cells or build sex hormones.

2. (*b*). If you don't smoke cigarettes, 220 isn't bad. But it is cause for concern. Current wisdom on cholesterol is "the lower the better." The ideal range is 130 to 190. Once your level of cholesterol goes above 200, your risk of heart disease rises rapidly. A level of 250 carries twice the risk of 200. For smokers, the numbers are harsher: 220 would be cause for alarm, since it is considered roughly equivalent to a level of 275 in a nonsmoker.

3. True in most cases. In light of the fact that you work out, don't smoke, and aren't overweight, the occasional steak is probably a forgivable indulgence (although beef is high in cholesterol and saturated fats). Exercise has been shown to raise the blood levels of high-density lipoproteins, or HDL's, which flush cholesterol from the body.

4. (*b*). High-density lipoproteins are fats that capture cholesterol and remove it from the body. Men have lower levels of HDL than women, which may explain why women have 60 percent fewer heart attacks than men. The normal blood level for HDL is 36 to 59.

5. False. A recent Harvard Medical School study showed that men between the ages of 20 and 60 who exhibited a high risk of developing heart disease were able to add as much as 12 months to their life expectancy by switching to a low-fat, low-cholesterol diet. Studies with rhesus monkeys have shown that a low-cholesterol diet reduced the occlusion of their arteries from 60 percent to 20 percent. Your arteries may not return to their original diameter, but you can still benefit from eliminating high-cholesterol foods.

6. (*b*). Americans consume as much as five times the optimal amount of cholesterol per day. There is clearly room for improvement. In societies where the population consumes only about 100 milligrams of cholesterol per day, heart disease rarely occurs.

7. (*c*). Foods such as cheese and meat contain both cholesterol and fat. On the other hand, egg yolks and shellfish are low in fat but high in cholesterol. By contrast, coconut oil and peanut butter have lots of fat but no cholesterol. The best rule of thumb for cholesterol watchers is this: Animal foods contain cholesterol, but vegetable foods do not.

8. False. Very few people—only about one in 500—have a genetic flaw that retards the removal of cholesterol from their blood and dooms them to developing heart disease. For most people, diet is a far more important factor.

9. (*b*). Egg yolks, liver, and ice cream are among the greatest sources of cholesterol in our diet. Mayonnaise is a villain because it contains egg yolks, and coconut oil is high in saturated fats. By contrast, low-fat cottage cheese, egg whites, and fish such as tuna are low in cholesterol. Vegetables and grains do not contain cholesterol. Baked goods are high in cholesterol only when they contain butter and eggs.

10. (*c*). Ranch is the least of three evils. Mayonnaise contains cholesterol, but buttermilk is made from skim milk and has very little cholesterol. To further minimize the cholesterol in your salad dressing, ask for ranch with low-fat yogurt instead of mayonnaise. Even better, dress your salad with olive oil and vinegar.

11. (*b*). There's considerable debate over whether eggs are an excellent food or something to be avoided. There is no question that one egg contains about twice the recommended daily intake of cholesterol, all of it in the yolk. If you have a high cholesterol count, consider giving up egg yolks. Egg whites contain no cholesterol and can be used in baking.

12. False. Contrary to popular belief, bypass surgery does not produce a "new you." Surgery doesn't address the root cause of heart disease, and it doesn't prevent future hardening of the arteries. The blood vessels that are transplanted from the legs to the heart are just as vulnerable to atherosclerosis as the old ones. Surgery is only a temporary—and very expensive—answer to advanced heart disease.

13. (*a*). Men under 40 with all three of these major risk factors are often among the 600,000 or so Americans who die of heart disease every year. It appears that smoking, high blood pressure, and high cholesterol are all about equally dangerous risk factors for heart disease.

14. (*c*). Cholesterol levels change relatively slowly. Frequent tests for it are unnecessary. The American Heart Association recommends that healthy men under 60 have their cholesterol checked every 5 years; between 60 and 75, every 2½ years; and yearly therafter.

How to Score

Give yourself 7 points for each correct multiple-choice answer and 6 points for each correct true/false answer. The maximum score is 94.

If you scored 80 to 94 points, congratulations. You are probably either a research biologist or a registered dietitian. You are already capable of controlling your cholesterol level and risk of heart disease entirely on your own.

A score of 60 to 79 points is good, but there's plenty of room for improvement. Keep a diary of the foods you eat for a couple of days. Record the number of times you eat eggs, cheese, or beef. Scan the list of ingredients of packaged foods for coconut oil or egg yolks.

If your score was 32 to 59 points, it's time to go on cholesterol alert. Your refrigerator is undoubtedly full of butter, Brie, eggs, Omaha steak and Swedish ice cream. Begin reading more about heart disease and diet. Take up regular aerobic exercise.

At 0 to 32 points, you might consider dialing 911. Better yet, contact your friends. Gather them together. Instead of talking about wine, the stock market, and compact disks, discuss cholesterol. It's a topic that should be near and dear to your heart.

Weight-Loss Updates

Shape-Up Secrets from the Slimming Pros

Will today be your day to decide once and for all to slim down and shape up? If so, it's time to lay the groundwork—planning your strategies, lining up your support systems, removing all those mental obstacles. In fact, say the experts, this headwork is crucial to the long-term success of any bodywork program. Here, then, is an enticing selection of smart "head starts" from America's top better-body pros—people who've built their reputations on helping others get in shape.

Jake Steinfeld

The 6′1″, 236-pound driving force behind the "Body By Jake" empire, which includes a celebrity fitness-training service, New York City health club, a daily exercise segment for cable television, exercise videos and a book entitled, of course, *Body by Jake,* offers these tips.

● Ease into exercise. One sure way to set yourself up for dropping out is to jump into a 1½ hour workout program. Instead, start with 5 minutes one day, 9 the next, and 12 after that until you eventually reach a half hour.
● Hang a smashing dress or other article of clothing (sized for the slimmer you) next to your mirror and look at it when you get dressed in the morning. Then try it on about once a week for motivation.

● Don't eat after 7:00 P.M. The calories from late-night dinners tend to stick. Morning meals, on the other hand, have all day to burn off.

● Don't fight the urge to throw in the towel. Play along. Let's say, for example, you feel like quitting 15 minutes into your half-hour walk. Tell yourself, "Okay, I quit," and start for home. Chances are you will change your mind and go the distance.

I use this strategy with clients. When I say, "Now give me 50 sit-ups!" and they ask if they can just do 20, I'll say, "Fine." Rarely does anyone stop short of 50.

Deborah Szekely

Here are suggestions from the founder and owner of one of the most luxurious health spas in the world, the Golden Door in Escondido, California, and its sister spa, Rancho La Puerta in Tecate, Mexico (Baja California).

● Think of food as units of energy. Got a pretty sedentary day in store? Eat lightly; you'll require less fuel. Got a tennis match or a five-mile hike scheduled? Stoke your furnace with complex carbohydrates.

● Eat for your health, not for your figure. Avoid restricted low-calorie diets. Not only will your health suffer but chances are, you'll gain back the lost weight. Concentrate instead on a healthy, low-fat, high-carbohydrate diet. By eating with your health in mind, you'll not only feel better, you'll gradually but permanently lose that excess weight.

● Find an object that weighs what you want to lose and carry it around for a little while. You'll quickly realize what a burden this excess weight is to your body. Even ten extra pounds means a significant amount of stress. You can visualize this and get the same impact. Imagine, for example, that for every extra pound of fat, your body has to support some 20 more miles of blood vessels.

● Think "movement" from dawn to dusk. Our ancestors had a natural pattern of movement. They gathered firewood, carried water, hunted on foot, worked the land. Movement was central to their existence; they didn't have to think about it. We do.

● Keep up your circle of friends. They are the best substitute for unnecessary food. If you are happy, you are less inclined to overeat.

● Don't feel obligated to clean your plate when dining out. The typical restaurant portion is designed with a 5'8", average, active man in mind. *You* don't need this much food. Cut back.

● Ask yourself: What will my later years be like? Active, exciting, healthy? Or sedentary, boring, and unhealthy? You can determine that with exercise and a diet of healthy foods and thoughts. And the time to do it is *now.*

Jack La Lanne

The man who has been "America's Fitness King" for 50 years, 30 of them on national daily television, has lots of pointers for exercise and weight loss. Here is a sampling.

● Revamp your exercise program every two weeks—not just to prevent monotony but also to ensure that your muscles are getting a well-rounded workout.

● Don't let your age get in the way of your aspirations. You can always improve your body and your health. A 90-year-old woman just starting to exercise won't be able to look like a 16-year-old, but she'll be the sexiest 90-year-old around!

● Take your measurements or a Polaroid photo of yourself every two weeks. Seeing progress will motivate you.

● Expect to pay some dues, at least in the beginning. Exercise is hard work. It's tough. Sometimes it hurts. Don't get discouraged. The payoff is worth it.

● Earn the right to do something "bad." Want to eat a 400-calorie dessert at dinner tonight? Go ahead. Just make sure you burn 650 calories through exercise to compensate.

● If you're out of shape, there's only one butt to kick, and that's yours. Don't blame it on the fact that you gave birth to three kids or have a sedentary desk job. Take responsibility for your weight and your health.

Art Mollen, D.O.

Dr. Mollen, director of the Southwest Health Institute in Phoenix, Arizona, and author of *The Mollen Method: A*

30-Day Program to Lifetime Health Addiction, offers the following suggestions.

● Exercise in the morning. By evening, you've found too many excuses to skip it. I've studied my patients and found that 75 percent of those who exercise in the morning stick with it. Afternoon exercisers have a 50 percent compliance rate. And only 25 percent of those who say they'll work out in the evening actually get around to it.

● If you're trying to sell yourself an excuse for not working out on a particular day, at least do half of what you had originally intended.

● Don't set yourself up for a bad exercise experience. Wait at least three hours after a meal to work out. If you eat too close to your exercise time, not enough blood will be able to get to your muscles because it'll be tied up in your stomach digesting your meal. Possible consequences are cramps and diarrhea.

Linda Crawford and Sadie Drumm

Here's advice from the behavioral specialist and exercise physiologist at Green Mountain at Fox Run, a Vermont-based center for weight and health management. Together, they've achieved an enviable success record; according to one study, nearly 50 percent of their clients maintain or better their weight loss five years later. Most programs see only about a 10 percent success rate after a year.

● Stop postponing life "until you're thin." Buy new clothes, change your hairstyle, join that aerobics class *now*. Once you start feeling better about the way you look, you'll be more motivated to tackle a weight problem. It's harder to slim down when you're depressed.

● Think of the urge to eat as a suggestion, not a command. A command is an order; you'll feel at the mercy of food. A suggestion gives you a choice. When you choose not to eat that snack, you gain confidence that you can indeed be in charge of your body.

● Fill your cookie jar with slips of paper that have enjoyable activities written on them, such as "buy flowers for the kitchen table" or "write a letter to a friend." Then, when the urge to binge or snack hits, steal a calorie-free surprise from the cookie jar.

● Don't lose sight of your "thin and fit" benefits and your "fat and out-of-shape" consequences. As a reminder, jot them down on an index card. On one side, list all the reasons why you want to slim down, such as "I want to shop anywhere and know I will find clothes that fit me," or "I hate being out of breath when I climb stairs."

On the other side, list the consequences of overeating and not exercising, such as "I have no energy," or "I no longer feel comfortable wearing my blouses tucked in." Keep a copy of the card in your desk, wallet or purse and car for easy reference.

● Going to a restaurant or party? Plan your strategy ahead of time. It might be to order a low-fat entrée, skip dessert, or have only one alcoholic drink. Assess your performance when you leave. Did you stick to your plan? Can you do it again?

● Try this high-impact graphic motivator: Pick a destination on a map and calculate its distance from your home. Then set out to exercise your way there. Record the number of miles you walk, run, swim, or bike each day. Plan a special celebration when you "reach" your destination.

● Don't weigh yourself. Notice instead how your clothes fit, how flexible your body's getting, the drop in your resting and recovering heart rates, the gains you've made in your strength and endurance. The truth is, it's possible to drop down two clothing sizes and not lose a pound. So if you're plotting your progress by the scale, you may unjustly see yourself as a failure.

● Make a dozen "exercise connections." That is, think of ways to connect familiar (but passive) activities with exercise. Walk to a newspaper stand instead of having the paper delivered. At work, deliver a memo by hand instead of sending it through interoffice mail.

● Make exercise convenient. Lay out your exercise clothes at night for morning workouts. Join a health club or aerobics club close to home or work, even if you have a slight preference for one on the other side of town. If getting to any club is too inconvenient, keep your walking shoes in tow and walk whenever you get the chance.

● Encourage your spouse or partner to join you in your healthful pursuits. You can support each other and share the satisfaction of achieving your goals.

Suzann Johnson

Johnson, a registered dietitian who is nutritionist for Weight Watchers International, recommends the following methods.

● Make sure you're really ready to trim down. Remember, you can't succeed without commitment. The desire and commitment must come from *you*, not your spouse or a friend who is needling you to lose weight.
● Choose a weight-loss program that makes sense to you. The worst thing is to follow a crazy fad diet just because a friend or splashy advertisement claims it's great.
● Make gift-giving (and receiving) fitness oriented. Ballroom dance lessons, tennis court time, or a spa membership are ideal presents.
● The next time you have a party, break out of the cake-and-punch or sit-down-dinner mold. Get together and have a sledding or skating party, a square dance, or a picnic with softball and Frisbee instead.
● If you stray off course—say, you don't exercise for five days straight, for example—don't think, "Oh, now I've ruined everything. I have to start over." The benefits of those weeks of diligence haven't been wiped out. Just don't overdo to make up for lost time. Take it easy to prevent injuries.

Sheila Cluff

And finally, some words of wisdom from the owner and director of two California health and fitness spas (the Oaks at Ojai and the Palms at Palm Springs) and author of *Sheila Cluff's Aerobic Body Contouring,* who is a true inspiration at 51 (5′4″, 102 pounds).

● Don't go hungry. Believe it or not, people can have trouble losing weight because they don't eat *enough*. When you take in too few calories, your metabolism slows in an attempt to prevent starvation.

Just make sure to choose your foods wisely. Vegetables

and whole grains should nudge your metabolism without piling the weight on. And remember: Don't eat fewer than 1,000 calories a day unless you're under a doctor's supervision or at a health spa. Spas generally make every bite of food count nutritionally.

● Make exercise an integral part of your daily life, like eating. Schedule it at a convenient time every day. If something occasionally interferes with your exercise time, don't worry. Everyone skips lunch now and then, too.

● Get an exercise buddy. You'll feel obligated to work out if someone else is depending on you.

● Once you're comfortable with the workout you've chosen, plan to add some resistance. Wear light wrist or ankle weights, or try one of the new waist belts with small weight bars you can add one at a time.

The Weight-Loss Guide to Kitchen Design

Food is tempting—everybody knows that. But did it ever occur to you that the place you keep your food could be tempting you, too? Take a look around your kitchen. The cookie jar in the corner is no dieter's friend. Those canisters of sugar, flour, and cocoa that you stare at every morning over your coffee cup almost beg you to "turn us into homemade cookies."

Your kitchen need not be a standing invitation to overeat or to cook less-than-wholesome food. Here's a way to slim your kitchen as you slim yourself.

First, clear your counters of nonnutritious foods and ingredients. Next, take a look at these ideas for stocking your kitchen for preparing healthier, leaner food. You don't have to spend a lot of money on new equipment, since you probably already have some of these items. You can always buy the others gradually. Before you know it, you'll have a new kitchen to go along with your new outlook on eating. These tools will make slim, healthy cooking a breeze—almost as easy as slipping on your new, slim clothes.

Hot-Air Popcorn Popper ● No oil goes into this electric popcorn maker, which can turn out a hot, wholesome and low-calorie snack in a matter of minutes. And it takes up a lot less room than a can of pretzels or potato chips!

Blender ● Its multiple functions make it practical to have on hand, especially for puréeing vegetables into "cream" soups without the cream.

Oven Bags ● For use in both conventional and microwave ovens, these bags create a moist environment—without added fats—to keep lean meats and poultry from drying out during cooking.

Bowl of Fruit ● You can put this where the cookie jar used to be. If your hand automatically goes in that direction when you're hungry, you'll end up with something nutritious and low in calories to munch on.

Garlic ● In addition to its ability to perk up a bland dish without adding calories, garlic has amazing health benefits. To maintain optimum firmness and flavor, store garlic in a dark, airy spot at about 50°F.

Slow Cooker ● The leanest cuts of meat often require the longest cooking. With a slow cooker you add the ingredients, plug it in, and leave for work or shopping. When you get home, the meal is done.

Double Boiler ● Yes, this utensil is good for more than melting chocolate. It helps warm up leftovers, like potatoes, vegetables, or meat casseroles, without butter or oil. It also is handy in making the lighter sauces that are part of the slim cook's repertoire.

Egg Coddler ● Weight-conscious cooks know that eggs are best boiled in water, not fried in fat. Now, for an easy and tasty alternative to soft-boiled or poached, try coddled eggs. Just break open your egg into a ceramic coddler, toss in an assortment of fresh herbs and a grind of pepper, twist on the lid, and gently simmer for about 6 minutes. Voilá—a perfectly cooked egg that's not only easy to prepare, it's easy to eat right out of its pretty coddler.

Fish Poacher ● For anyone but the true fish lover, this piece of equipment is indeed extravagant. But if you catch your own or buy fish fresh and whole, you might want to consider a poacher to enjoy your fish the way the Europeans do—delicately cooked with herbs and vegetables in a poaching liquid.

Food Processor ● This handy device can do just about everything a blender can do and more. It cuts, chops, grates, and juliennes vegetables within seconds. Of course, you burn fewer calories chopping this way than you would with the manual method. But some claim that the food processor's fine cutting action releases juices, particularly from onions, that reduce the need for butter or oil in sautéing.

Grains and Legumes ● Fill your canisters with a variety of grains. Split peas, millet, lentils, beans, and a wide variety of whole wheat pastas will give you a dried-foods pantry at the ready.

Fresh Herbs ● To make the most of your slim-foods cooking, keep a supply of fresh herbs on your kitchen windowsill. Dried just can't match the taste of, say, fresh basil with summer tomatoes. You'll never miss the oily dressing!

Nonstick Pans ● Today they come in all sizes and shapes and price ranges. The advantage? They allow you to sauté without the addition of any fat. Every weight watcher should have at least one.

Wooden Spoons ● Essential to protect nonstick pans from scratches when you're cooking without fat.

Nonstick Spray ● When you're sautéing, even a nonstick pan can benefit from a quick "spritz" of nonstick spray. Made from lecithin, it can "grease" a pan with just 7 calories. That, compared to a tablespoon of oil or butter at about 100 calories.

Ridged Cast-Iron Skillet ● For flash-in-the-pan cooking without the grease, this handy tool is great for grilling boneless chicken breasts or even sirloin burgers. The ridges help capture excess fat and keep it off your food.

Clay Cooker ● Another utensil perhaps only the serious cook can appreciate, the clay cooker allows meats to simmer slowly in their own juices, making the use of extra fats, sauces or broths unnecessary.

Kitchen Scale ● Is that really a three-ounce portion of fish you're serving yourself? When in doubt, lay it out—on your handy kitchen food scale. It's a tool that's indispensable when trying to keep your calories in check. One buying tip: Look for a diet scale that's sensitive to the quarter ounce—usually, one with a maximum one-pound reading.

Skimmer and Gravy Strainer ● To improve the low-calorie goodness of soups, stews and gravies, try these gadgets. A flat, mesh skimmer easily removes cold, congealed fat from the top of soups and stews, and the pitcherlike gravy strainer allows you to separate fat from hot broth and gravy.

Spaghetti Measurer ● Pasta is great diet food, but not when you eat it by the pound. How many times have you made spaghetti and wound up with enough to wind around your kitchen—twice? This inexpensive little device guarantees you'll cook the right amount.

Steamer ● Whether you choose a simple stainless-steel basket or an elaborate multitiered oriental bamboo variety, a steamer is perfect for cooking vegetables to perfection—al dente.

Strainer ● Use this to rinse all the fresh fruits and vegetables you'll have on hand. In fact, you'll use it so often, you might want to have two or three, in different sizes, of course.

Wok ● Stir-frying is a great way to cook. While a little fat is required, you don't need nearly the amount that is required for pan-frying. And as your wok gets seasoned with use, you'll find you can get away with using less and less.

Microwave Oven ● Since microwaves cook with moist heat, there's no need to use butter or oil to prevent food from sticking to dishes. Microwaving also preserves important vitamins and minerals sometimes lost with other cooking methods. The result: better nutrition and fewer calories.

Vinegar ● That's right, no oil. Just vinegar. Vinegar can stand alone quite well on a salad. And with the tasty variety of flavored vinegars on the market today, you might be able to find some pretty bottles to start a collection. Raspberry, balsamic and tarragon are a nice trio to start with.

Those Last Ten Pounds: How to Nudge the Unbudgeable

Nearly everyone's got 'em. Stubborn pounds. The kind that quietly creep up over the years and seemingly settle in for life. Diet-resistant, they hang on after the other unwanted pounds have gone. And once pried from your frame, they are almost certain to return as quickly as they came off. To make matters worse, it's usually the last ten pounds that put you within striking distance of your weight goal that are least likely to surrender without a fight. But why should the last ten be any tougher to shed than the first?

"I'll give you three simple reasons," says Theodore Van

Itallie, M.D., codirector of the Division of Metabolism and Nutrition at St. Luke's/Roosevelt Hospital in New York City. "First, fatter people tend to have higher energy requirements. As you lose weight, you burn fewer calories just by virtue of the fact that you've become smaller and are carrying around less weight. Second, heavy people tend to be waterlogged, and water loss is the first thing to show up on the scale. Third, as you lose weight, your metabolic rate slows down."

The Lose/Gain Merry-Go-Round

Rapid weight loss and weight cycling—rapid weight loss followed by rapid weight gain—exacerbate the problem. Eating too little can sometimes sabotage your weight-loss efforts, Dr. Van Itallie explains. When denied food, the body feeds off the protein in muscle. And since muscle is the body's most metabolically active tissue, depleting it can reduce your body's calorie-burning ability.

Further, according to George L. Blackburn, M.D., Ph.D., associate professor at Harvard Medical School and a leading authority on weight loss, a severely restricted diet trains the body to be more energy efficient—that is, to conserve calories by slowing its resting metabolic rate. This, he says, makes it increasingly difficult to continue losing weight and much easier to gain it back, since the metabolism usually stays depressed even after normal eating patterns resume.

Regained weight is especially stubborn. The problem is, crash dieting not only depletes muscle mass, it promotes fat storage later, after you've gone off the diet. So pounds lost as muscle are often regained as fat. Preliminary studies have shown that as weight loss/gain cycling progresses (and the body's percentage of fat may increase), weight loss occurs more slowly and regain occurs more rapidly. "This may be why losing becomes more difficult as we get older. The body learns from many bouts of dieting, and stores fat in preparation for another shortage," says Kelly Brownell, Ph.D., codirector of the obesity research group at the University of Pennsylvania School of Medicine.

Still, dietmongers insist that the more resistant the weight problem, the more drastic the measures required to resolve it.

The experts we interviewed disagree with that: Stubborn pounds, they say, eventually yield to gentle persuasion. The person who takes a slow and steady approach may have a much better chance of dropping those last ten pounds permanently.

Their general advice: Forget about extremely restricted diets or strenuous exercise regimens. What's required is patience and commitment. Don't tackle a tough weight problem unless you are quite motivated and are certain that you can stick with the kind of lifestyle changes mentioned below—not just till you've shed the ten pounds but forever, for the rest of your life.

"Look at it this way," says Dr. Van Itallie. "You can lose weight by moving from New York City to Bangladesh for two months. But when you move back to New York City you'll gain it right back. The key is to learn to live in your New York environment at a different level of energy intake and expenditure—at a different calorie economy."

Advice from the Experts

So, if you are motivated and committed, the experts are ready to share their strategies for permanent weight loss. Here are the recommendations of Dr. Van Itallie, Dr. Blackburn, and Dr. Brownell for three common "stubborn-pound" scenarios.

Suppose, over the last five years, your weight has stabilized at a level ten pounds above your ideal. You eat sensibly, consuming about 1,600 to 1,800 calories a day, and exercise regularly—30 minutes, three times a week. How can you safely shed those ten pounds and maintain the lower weight?

"The best way to lose fat and retain lean muscle mass is to lose weight slowly. You can do this by reducing caloric intake by about 500 calories per day and gradually increasing caloric expenditure through exercise," says Dr. Van Itallie. "Safe weight loss occurs at an average rate of 1 percent of body weight per week. If you weigh 150 pounds, for example, aim for a loss of about 1½ pounds a week, no more."

Dr. Blackburn's advice is similar. "If you've got ten pounds to lose, give it a full ten weeks," he says. "In the first three to four weeks, you can expect to lose half the weight. In the next four weeks, you lose a pound a week. And in the last two weeks you'll shape up and lose more fat.

"Keep in mind that your ideal weight is one you can maintain without being hungry while eating three natural meals a day," he adds. "So don't starve yourself. Eat. Just pare down your diet to the essentials—the raw materials. Whole-wheat bread. Pasta. Rice. Fruits and vegetables. Skim milk. Fish and skinless chicken. No mixed dishes. No goulash. No lasagna."

By eating a "raw-materials diet," as Dr. Blackburn calls it, you consume more complex carbohydrates and less fat. The most obvious advantage of this diet is that it satisfies by providing bulk. More important, it gives your weight-loss program a metabolic edge.

Calories from fat are metabolized quickly and efficiently. In other words, it takes very little energy to transform butter into body fat. Calories from carbohydrates present the body with a greater challenge. It takes about five times as much energy to store the calories from, say, bread, than it does from butter.

Of course, to burn calories, trim body fat, build muscle, regulate appetite, and ensure weight-loss success, exercise also plays a crucial role. Especially the right kind.

"You have to make a distinction between exercise that is designed for cardiovascular fitness and exercise that is designed for weight loss," says Dr. Van Itallie. "Thirty minutes of aerobic exercise three times a week will improve your cardiovascular condition. But for significant weight loss, I recommend gradually working up to two hours of brisk, purposeful walking every day. For maintenance, you can cut back to about an hour a day."

Dr. Blackburn agrees that, if you're exercising to lose weight, frequency and duration take precedence over intensity. "Instead of a strenuous aerobic regimen three times per week, I'd suggest a more moderate routine—say, walking or bicycling— five to seven days a week," he says. Of course, the more time you can devote to exercise the better. But to be realistic, he says, most people would do well if they could walk for 40 minutes a day.

Suppose you've embarked on a low-calorie diet and shed 25 to 30 pounds as a result. The weight came off pretty fast. But the diet doesn't seem to be working anymore. You've stalled 10 pounds from your weight goal. How do you get past this plateau?

First, say the experts, congratulate yourself. A 30-pound weight loss is worth celebrating. Reward yourself with a vacation—a vacation from weight loss. That's not to say, binge back the 30 pounds. Rather, ease up to a maintenance plan.

If you've just dropped a fast 30 pounds, chances are you're in a very different metabolic state than you were before dieting, Dr. Van Itallie explains. The challenge now is to stabilize yourself at the new weight. If you're able to do this for a few months, your body should be better prepared to let go of the last 10 pounds.

Dr. Brownell seconds this "vacation" strategy. "Last year I had the opportunity to meet with a large group of individuals who averaged a 100-pound weight loss. I asked them how they overcame their weight-loss plateaus. Several said that they took a break from dieting and maintained their losses for a period of time before they took up dieting again," he explains.

To maintain a lower weight, you can eat more than you did while dieting but less than you ate at the higher weight.

"Keep in mind that for every pound you lose, you will burn 10 calories less per day just because you are lighter," says Dr. Blackburn. "So, to maintain a 30-pound loss, you'll have to eat 300 calories a day less or burn 300 calories a day more than you did at your higher weight."

"You probably have to change the nature of your diet, too, so that you're eating foods lower in fat and higher in complex carbohydrates," Dr. Van Itallie adds, "and adjust your lifestyle to make more room for exercise."

Only after you've maintained the 30-pound loss for at least three to six months should you tackle the last 10 pounds, the experts agreed. When you're ready, then, follow the advice given for the first scenario: Take it slow, eat a moderately reduced high-carbohydrate diet and gear yourself up for an hour or so of brisk walking every day.

Suppose you've repeatedly lost and gained ten pounds. Now, you're finding it virtually impossible to take them off again. What can you do to put an end to weight cycling and rid yourself of this unwanted weight once and for all?

"If you've lost before, this time you may have a more difficult battle to fight," says Dr. Brownell. "This doesn't mean that you won't lose this weight. But there is a possibility it's going to take more—more calorie cuts, more exercise and, most important, more motivation and commitment."

"People who continually regain their losses are obviously on the wrong track," says Dr. Van Itallie. "Those people have to take a careful look at their lifestyle and see whether, in fact, they are willing to commit themselves to permanent changes.

"Ask yourself: Am I really prepared to walk or bicycle one hour a day every day for the rest of my life? Am I really prepared to permanently give up fried foods, fatty meats and whole milk in favor of fruits, vegetables, fish, and other low-fat, high-fiber fare? If you can't answer yes, without hesitation, to those questions, then it's a waste of time, energy and emotion to lose those ten pounds. You'll only gain them back—again."

However (here's the best news) if you can answer with a resounding yes, your battle of the bulge is as good as won.

Dining Out on a Calorie Budget

What dieter doesn't suffer from "restaurant anxiety"—the crippling fear of blowing weeks of weight control in one madcap indulgence? Well, fear no more. With a little menu savvy, you can dodge and weave your way through just about any eatery and emerge with your waistline intact.

To help you do this, scores of menus from a wide array of restaurants were reviewed for the purpose of comparing calorie data. The discoveries may surprise you: There are lots of delightfully satisfying low-calorie choices, even at eateries that traditionally serve fattening fare. The recommendations that follow are based on U.S. Department of Agriculture calorie counts for standard servings. (Keep in mind that portions and recipes do vary widely from one eating establishment to another.)

Here then, the good, the bad, and the best dinner choices for the calorie conscious.

Seafood Restaurant

The restaurant of choice for many dieters, seafood houses sometimes serve up deceptively fattening fare. A dozen steamed clams doesn't sound like much. But dunked in butter, they can add up to nearly 300 calories. And that's just the appetizer.

Similarly, a "low-calorie" entrée like flounder stuffed with crabmeat can easily top 500 calories if it's smothered with white sauce. Beware, too, of seafood dishes with fancy last names, such as Lobster Newburg (725 calories) or Clams Casino (550). And steer clear of combination platters. These king-size dinners often feature fried fish and high-calorie concoctions such as deviled crab or crab cakes.

Better Alternatives ● Take tomato-based Manhattan clam chowder over the creamy New England version and save half the calories (about 80 per cup). For similar savings, choose a clear seafood gumbo over a smooth and creamy seafood bisque. Shrimp cocktail (at 100 calories for five large shrimp with cocktail sauce) is the obvious choice over steamed clams with butter. An eight-ounce lobster tail, at just 115 calories, or six steamed whole hardshell crabs, at 144, are fine dinner entrées if you can do without the butter. If you can't, stick to broiled white fish, such as flounder, scrod or haddock, moistened with lemon juice.

Best Bet ● "Pick and peel" shrimp with cocktail sauce. Beyond the obvious caloric advantage, any seafood—such as shrimp in the shell, stone-crab claws or steamed hardshell crabs—that you must first pry from its shell slows eating to an appetite-satisfying pace.

Our entrée recommendation is grilled kabob of shrimp, scallops, or white fish and vegetables at 230 calories per serving.

American Steak House

A juicy steak, the dieter's choice of years gone by, has fallen from favor. The reason: Many cuts of beef are high in fat, and fat is high in calories. Generally, the better the cut, the more calories from fat. Filet mignon, Delmonico, and New York strip steaks owe their tenderness to fat marbling. Beware, too, steak-house toppings such as mushrooms, onions, or peppers. They are usually sautéed in butter.

Better Alternatives ● From a calorie standpoint, London broil is a cut above the rest. At 477 calories for a generous (but often standard) eight-ounce portion, it contains up to 200 calories less per serving than the steaks mentioned above. Another calorie-miser tip: Order your meat cooked medium-well; the longer the meat cooks, the more fat is rendered from it.

Best Bet ● Cut your steak in half; offer the other half to your table partner or take it home for another meal. Then center your meal around other standard steak-house items: salad and baked potato. Ask for some low-calorie salad dressing on the side to sprinkle over your greens and potato (instead of sour cream or butter).

American Diner

Diners tend to serve many precooked dishes, such as meat loaf and chicken croquettes, that are loaded with fattening fillers. Made-to-order items are often grilled in grease or fried.

Better Alternatives ● Roast turkey, at 132 calories without gravy, or broiled haddock or flounder, at 117 without butter, are standard on almost every diner menu. Ordering mashed potatoes (without gravy or butter) instead of bread stuffing saves you another 200 calories. For an appetizer, choose a half grapefruit or a melon wedge (each less than 50 calories) over fruit cup, which may carry the extra weight of a sugary syrup. Or have a glass of tomato juice. At 21 calories, it has about half the caloric clout of orange or apple juice and less than one-fourth the calories of grape juice.

Best Bet ● Create a 1980s' grazing experience in a 1950s' diner setting. Order a tossed salad, dressing on the side, and an assortment of vegetables. Pickled cabbage, unsweetened apple-sauce, string beans, corn, and low-fat cottage cheese don't add up to a hill of beans, calorically speaking. But keep in mind that pickled red beets, at 90 calories a half-cup serving, are an unexpected heavy hitter.

Pizza Shop

Pizza alone is not bad: about 120 calories for a slice of a thin-crust pie. It's the toppings that can spell trouble. Just 4½ slices of pepperoni double the calories in a slice of pizza. Black olives and anchovies packed in oil also carry a hefty share of calories from fat.

Better Alternatives ● Top your pizza with fresh vegetables, such as onions, garlic, green and red peppers, and mushrooms. Go easy on the cheese and olive oil.

Best Bet ● One slice of thick-crust pizza, topped with all the veggies you can eat. At about 165 satisfying calories, it has half the cheese and about 100 calories less than two slices of vegetable-topped thin-crust pizza.

Delicatessen

Think "deli" and you probably conjure up an image of dining on the biggest hot pastrami sandwich you can possibly fit between your jaws. In reality, that can cost you upwards of 700 calories for six ounces of meat between two slices of rye. And, you haven't tackled the "help yourself" table full of pickles, potato salad, and coleslaw! Here, lunch can easily cost you your full day's allowance of calories, especially if you splurge on cheesecake for dessert.

Better Alternatives ● Take a friend and share a sandwich. Then "weigh" each sandwich ingredient alone and, more important, together. At 106 calories, three ounces of turkey meat, for example, is the clear choice over roast beef at 150. But when the roast beef is accompanied by mustard or horse-radish (each about 4 to 5 calories a tablespoon) and the drier turkey meat requires mayo or Russian dressing (100 and 75 calories, respectively), the scales tip in favor of the roast beef. Final score: half of a turkey sandwich, 267 calories; roast beef, 216. For extras, opt for pickled cabbage or a great big deli pickle, which won't cost you more than 10 calories. If you must indulge in dessert, choose a cheese blintz. Made with cottage cheese, it contains half as many calories as New York-style cheesecake (about 140).

Best Bet ● Half a deli sandwich consisting of three ounces of roast turkey, lettuce, tomato and mustard on one slice of rye (just 178 calories) or lox with tomato and onion on half a bagel (142).

Mexican Restaurant

South-of-the-border cuisine offers excellent diet fare, especially dishes that are light on meat and heavy on toppings like chopped tomato and pepper, shredded lettuce and salsa. There are two danger zones, however: fried foods and *grande* platter portions. An order of nachos (deep-fried tortilla chips topped with melted cheese and refried beans, often prepared with lard) will cost you about 800 calories. And there's more trouble in the main event: Entrées heaped high with guacamole, refried beans, cheese, and sour cream contain *mucho* calories.

Better Alternatives ● Order a la carte. Pass up the crisp corn tortillas (which are fried) and request soft flour tortillas (which are baked). Hold the cheese, sour cream, and guacamole for an additional calorie saving. And, instead of the lard-laden refried beans, take a side order of Mexican rice, worth about 50 calories less. Another smart choice: A bowl of chili with beans saves about 60 calories over the all-meat chili—hold the cheese, of course.

Best Bet ● A soft flour taco with chicken and rice, at just 300 calories, or a light burrito (soft flour tortilla filled with lettuce, tomato, chicken, and salsa), about 340.

Italian Restaurant

From simple spaghetti houses to fine Northern Italian restaurants, one caution applies: Watch out for olive oil. A tasty but fattening ingredient (at 120 calories per tablespoon), it lurks in the garlic bread, antipasto, pesto sauce, Caesar salad, roasted sweet peppers with anchovies or tuna, and much more. Another note on fine dining: If you're intent on doing as the Romans do, be prepared for the challenge of a five-course extravaganza.

Better Alternatives ● For starters, choose a cup of mine-strone (about 120 calories) or chicken broth with pasta (150) or an order of mussels with marinara sauce (120). Marinara, which is a meatless tomato sauce, and tomato-based red clam sauce are the lightest accompaniments to pasta. Served over a cup of spaghetti, they run about 250 calories. In the meat department, save calories by ordering chicken cacciatore, cooked in a tomato sauce, instead of chicken Parmesan, with breading and cheese. The veal dish of choice is picata, lightly sautéed with lemon. Finally, don't allow the waiter to sweet-talk you into cannoli, tortoni, or spumoni. Calorie-wise, these desserts vie with the best cakes and pies America has to offer. Even the Italian ice will cost you plenty: about 250 calories.

Best Bet ● For a five-course meal that comes in at around 500 calories, start with melon. Next, a cup of minestrone soup, then a green salad dressed with red-wine vinegar and a fresh grinding of black pepper. As an entrée, order an appetizer or child's portion of pasta with marinara sauce. Top the meal with fresh berries and a cup of espresso.

Chinese Restaurant

The Chinese restaurant has enjoyed a reputation for light food, and therein lies the danger. Calorie-conscious diners assume everything on the menu is safe for consumption. In fact, fried rice, fried noodles, fried wontons, and deep-fried egg rolls are heavyweights. Guess why.

Better Alternatives ● Choose chop suey over chow mein (which is traditionally served with fried noodles) for a 100-calorie-plus saving. Similarly, steamed rice is at least 50 calories less than fried rice. Hold the cornstarch for additional savings.

Best Bet ● Share an order of stir-fried chicken or shrimp with vegetables served over steamed rice.

French Restaurant

First the good news: Since the French pride themselves on freshly prepared food, it's very easy for the chef to customize a dish to your diet. Now the bad news: Coaxing low-calorie fare out of a classic French chef can be an exasperating task. Fortunately, heavy cream and butter sauces are giving way to the lighter nouvelle cuisine. If your chef seems stuck in the old ways, appeal to his sense of romance: Explain that your love life is inextricably linked to your waistline.

Better Alternatives ● Take *salade verte* (mixed greens) over *salade Niçoise* (greens mixed with olives, eggs, tuna, and anchovies) and save calories. Poached fish or quenelles (a poached fish dumpling of sorts made of pike and egg whites), or pot-au-feu (stewed chicken in broth) are excellent alternatives to the heavy, sauce-laden entrées. Know too that not all sauces are created equal: *coulis,* made of puréed vegetables, and *sauce piquante,* with tomatoes, vinegar, and shallots, are calorie-miles apart from *béarnaise* (with egg yolks and butter), *velouté* (butter, flour, and stock), *béchamel* (flour, butter, and milk),

SEVEN TIPS TO LIGHTEN UP YOUR DINNER ORDER

If eating out is a treat that you don't want to give up while on a weight-loss program, here are some more suggestions for calorie-conscious dining.

1. Scrutinize menu offerings with a keen eye for the two key diet destroyers: sugar and fat. Both concentrate calories.

2. Know not only what's in a dish but also how it's prepared. Frying foods can double the caloric count of an otherwise low-calorie food. Fried foods that are first breaded are particularly bad: The breading soaks up fat like a sponge. If "crispy" describes an item on the menu, don't give it a second glance: It's fried.

3. Keep meat to a minimum. By nature, meat is high in fat. Ironically, diet platters listed on many menus offer the hamburger without the bun. In fact, you're better off with just the bun.

4. Don't confuse healthy foods with low-calorie ones. Polyunsaturated oils and margarine may have a cholesterol-cutting edge over animal fats but, from a dieter's standpoint, they are as bad as butter. Similarly, fatty fish such as salmon and mackerel, which are considered especially good for the heart, can take your daily calorie count too far upstream.

5. Beware the salad bar. It's the little things that mean a lot. Croutons, sunflower seeds, chow mein noodles, bacon bits, and grated cheese pack even more calories per weight than the mayonnaise-based potato and macaroni salads. As for the dressings, oil and vinegar can be just as bad as the prepared blue cheese if you have a heavy hand with the oil.

6. Pare down portions. Limit your dinner choices to the appetizers. Or order your dinner family style; that is, one entrée, delivered to the center of the table, from which two people serve themselves.

7. Ask the waiter if he can recommend a low-calorie offering . . . but don't take his word for it. Waiters at a variety of restaurants were polled for such suggestions, with varying degrees of success.

and the crème de la crème, *Mornay,* made with béchamel sauce, heavy cream, egg yolks, and cheese.

Best Bet ● Bouillabaisse—*sans aioli* (without garlic mayonnaise). This tomato and saffron-flavored fish stew will keep you busy all night, prying mussels from their shells and lapping up every delicious drop of stock with French bread. A fabulous indulgence at just 450 calories, including the bread.

Body-Care Updates

Unwire Your High-Tension Zones

Is muscle tension creeping up on you? If a friend laid a hand on your shoulder right this minute, would the tightness there startle both of you?

Muscle tension affects people in a variety of ways. Some experience pain in their neck and shoulders. Others suffer from a tight jaw or tense back. Wherever you feel it, here's some practical help.

The Inside Story

Mental stress is a major cause of muscle tension. An infuriating phone call or family feud can prick your sympathetic nervous system into its well-known "fight or flight" response. Muscles tighten and stress hormones, such as adrenaline, are released. You feel uptight.

Usually, once the stress passes and the mind settles down, the physical symptoms subside: Hormones level off and clenched muscles relax. But, unfortunately, when *chronic* stress causes muscles to contract without release, blood vessels constrict, decreasing blood flow. "Lactic acid and other waste products like carbon dioxide accumulate," says Willibald Nagler, M.D., physiatrist-in-chief at New York Hospital-Cornell University Medical Center and author of *Dr. Nagler's Body Maintenance and Repair Book*. The muscles become starved for oxygen and signal their distress with pain.

Sometimes, a bundle of muscle fibers will contract suddenly and painfully, resulting in a muscle spasm. The nerves send loud pain messages to the brain, which responds by contracting the blood vessels. Until the affected muscle fibers relax and return to normal, movement and activity may be severely curtailed.

If muscle spasms are not released (through various forms of treatment), they can knot up into hard, tangled lumps called trigger points, notes Dr. Nagler. "Trigger points are an end result of prolonged muscle tightness," says Richard A. Fee, Ph.D., director of the psychophysiology research laboratory at the University of Louisville, Kentucky. Painful to the touch, they don't go away unless treated. Unfortunately, once trigger points develop, you're likely to get them again. "There is a tendency, once that kind of problem has developed, for it to become chronic," says Steven Fahrion, Ph.D., codirector of the voluntary controls program at the Menninger Foundation in Topeka, Kansas.

Not all muscle tension is caused by mental or emotional stress. Bad posture can result in cramping and eventual muscle fatigue. So can habitual positions that place undue stress on the muscles, such as hunching over a computer console for hours at a time. Diet may play a role. "There's a possibility that a chronic low-calcium diet may cause you to have muscle cramps," says William J. Evans, Ph.D., chief of the physiology laboratory at the U.S. Department of Agriculture Human Nutrition Research Center on Aging at Tufts University. A sedentary lifestyle can also be a factor in muscle tension. By sitting too much and moving too little, we effectively eliminate a simple and natural tension reliever: exercise.

Treats for a Tense Body

"The body is designed to release tension through exercise," says Emmett E. Miller, M.D., a California physician who specializes in stress-related problems. The healthy muscle contraction and release produced by a good game of tennis or a long walk helps muscles move past a contracted state. "It's hard for your muscles to stay tense if they've been tired out by repeated contractions," explains Paul D. Thompson, M.D., director of the cardiac rehabilitation program at Miriam Hospital and associate professor of medicine at Brown University.

Exercises that gently stretch muscles, keeping you limber, are a vital complement to brisk walking or other aerobic exercise. By keeping muscles relaxed, you help prevent the development of spasms and trigger points, notes Dr. Fahrion. Hatha-yoga, which consists of slow, gentle stretching, can be a real friend to tight muscles. (Caution: Stretching is not recommended for muscle spasms—it can make matters worse.)

Of course, anything that helps relieve stress can help prevent muscle tension. That includes meditation, progressive relaxation, visualization, and selective awareness exercises that can help put you in touch with your body's tension or pain signals. Biofeedback training can be useful both to prevent the buildup of muscle tension and as an "on-the-spot" method to relieve pain, says Dr. Fahrion.

Massage can loosen and relax tense muscles by sending more blood their way. "Massage should feel good and should leave you feeling good afterward," says Dr. Fee. Sometimes, however, if you are very tense and have well-established trigger points, touching can result in pain and spasm. Also, massage can aggravate an injury, trauma, or inflamed area. Solution: a licensed massage therapist who will explore your medical history before laying a hand on you.

Soothing the Zones

Here's a head-to-toe checklist with help for each trouble spot. *Note:* Tension-relieving exercises should be performed in a slow, purposeful way, while focusing on breathing. A rushed, distracted attitude only perpetuates the tension, says Jon Kabat-Zinn, Ph.D., assistant professor of preventive and behavioral medicine at the University of Massachusetts Medical School.

Head ● For many, the gripping pain of a tension headache signals the culmination of a bad day. But doctors are still unsure how these headaches take hold. "Some people theorize that maybe the tension is in the scalp muscles, but the true cause of tension headaches is difficult to decide," says Edward J. Resnick, M.D., professor of orthopedic surgery and director of the pain control center at the Temple University School of Medicine and Hospital. "They may be associated with emotional tension." The most common type of headache, tension headaches are "relatively benign," he says—small comfort when your head is throbbing.

Relief: If you can, lie down and rest or nap. Place a cool, damp washcloth across your forehead. Some people find that pressing the midpoint of each eyebrow helps to relieve headache pain. Any of the three common over-the-counter pain relievers—aspirin, acetaminophen, and ibuprofen—should help to quell a tension headache. Or ask your doctor to prescribe a nonnarcotic pain reliever or muscle relaxant.

Prevention: Biofeedback and relaxation techniques seem to help keep tension headaches at bay. And with practice, says Dr. Fahrion, you will be able to relax away a headache!

Face ● Surprisingly, a lot of tension-making activities take place here. If you frown while you read or concentrate, you're activating the "corrugator" muscle located above the bridge of your nose, says Dr. Fahrion. And every time you scowl, wrinkle your face or grimace, the facial muscles tighten. "The facial muscles are very vulnerable to the influence of emotions and they tighten up very easily," says Dr. Nagler.

Relief: "Be aware of tension in the facial musculature and the placement of the joints in your jaw," says Dr. Fee. Are your teeth touching? They shouldn't be, unless you're chewing. Where is your tongue? It should be resting comfortably in your mouth, pressed neither too far up nor too far down. If you find any telltale signs of tension, take a deep breath and let it out slowly.

Prevention: As in any tension zone, the first step is awareness. Is your forehead tense? Smooth a piece of Scotch tape horizontally across it and go about your business. Every time you scrunch your muscles, the pull of the tape will give you feedback.

Jaw ● Unlike the facial muscles, which are relatively delicate, the masseter muscle, which opens and closes the jaw, can pack a wallop. Like all joints in the body, the jaw rests on a "pad" of cartilage. "If your jaw muscles are always tight, you wear away the cartilage," says Dr. Nagler.

Jaw tension, along with clenching and grinding of the teeth, can radiate outward, causing headaches, earaches, and dull, aching facial pain along with tenderness of the jaw muscles —symptoms of temporomandibular joint (TMJ) disorders.

Relief: To ease mild jaw tightness, try a gentle stretch. "Open your mouth wide without forcing the jaw and inhale. Exhale slowly as you close your mouth, lightly massaging the muscles over the jaw hinge," suggests Gene Arbetter, Chicago massage therapist and spokesman for the American Massage Therapy Association. If you experience severe clenching, grinding or pain, see your dentist or doctor. Along with providing relief of symptoms and pain, your dentist may suggest wearing an orthodontic appliance during sleep.

Prevention: If the tension is caused by stress, relaxation techniques can help. Because TMJ can also be caused or worsened by a bad bite, dental work and orthodontics may be necessary to resolve the tension.

Neck ● Be kind to your neck. As you turn your head, the muscles in your neck alternately contract and relax, normally allowing for easy and painless movement. "The neck balances everything," says Dr. Nagler. "Therefore it's very vulnerable to tightening of the muscles if we are tense."

Relief: Mild cramps can probably be relieved by rest, massage, and gentle limbering, notes Dr. Nagler: Place left elbow in right hand, pull it over to the right side. Hold, then relax. Reverse. Next, place hands flat on your chest, palms down, elbows out to sides. Circle elbows forward and backward. Repeat three times. Do this several times a day, as often as tension occurs.

First aid for severe muscle spasms: Apply a cold pack or ice. "For acute muscle spasms, cold is much more soothing than heat," says Dr. Nagler. (Dr. Resnick suggests wrapping ice cubes or a fistful of crushed ice in a terry washcloth to keep your skin from freezing. Massage the painful area for five to ten minutes.) Pain causes nerves to contract the blood vessels. By numbing the nerves with cold, you quiet the pain messages, allowing your blood vessels to dilate and deliver blood to the besieged area. Cold performs a second useful function: It reduces fluid buildup in the muscle, a potential source of pressure around the spasm. After 48 hours, heat is more beneficial.

Next step: See a doctor. Dr. Nagler often treats neck spasms with gentle electrical stimulation "designed to mimic the natural contraction/relaxation pattern of your muscles," he says. The final stage of treatment: gentle, slow movement of the tight muscle—limbering and loosening, but never stretching it. "Limbering helps restore normal circulation and eases your fibers back into their customary patterns of contraction and relaxation," he says.

Prevention: Avoid vigorous neck rolls. "Full-circle or abrupt rotation of any part of the spine isn't kind to the disks, so neck rolls are falling out of favor," says Arbetter. Also, be conscious of your neck's position at all times and try to modify stressful activities. Instead of bending your neck to cradle the telephone, for example, hold the receiver with your hand and keep your neck upright, advises Arbetter. If you like to read in bed, sit up straight with your neck and spine aligned rather than at a 90-degree angle. You can ease your neck at night, too. Sleep on your back, using a rolled towel to support your neck. Rest your head on a low pillow or directly on the mattress.

Shoulders ● Many people experience shoulder tension. And, almost always, it's combined with tightness in the neck. Why are the shoulders such a common tension zone? "The phrase that we use, 'weight of the world on his shoulders,' has a lot of bearing in physical reality," says Arbetter. He theorizes that the shoulders represent our "shield" against a stressful world. Whatever the reason, we seem to tighten them every chance we get. We hunch behind the wheel. We shrug them during conversation. In cold weather, we even use our shoulders as earmuffs!

Relief: For mild shoulder tension, heat can be very soothing. "Moist heat is more penetrating than dry heat," says Dr. Nagler. Take a hot shower, or soak in a hot bath or Jacuzzi. "A home spa or whirlpool is a really good investment," says Dr. Fee. Rubdown ointments are another way to deliver warmth. They work by dilating the blood vessels, thereby delivering more oxygen to muscles. Warning: Never apply heat in conjunction with products containing menthol and methyl salicylate—the combination can result in severe internal damage.

For severe muscle spasms, follow the advice described for neck spasms: During the first 48 hours after injury, apply cold packs for 15 to 20 minutes at a time. After 48 hours, switch to heat treatments. See a doctor.

Trigger points often appear in the shoulders, notes Dr. Nagler. To force the clumped-up fibers apart, he injects them with saline fluid. Electrical stimulation, limbering exercises and, later on, stretching and strengthening exercises can help to resolve the condition.

Prevention: To keep shoulder muscles loose and relaxed, Dr. Kabat-Zinn recommends this mini-workout: Roll your shoulders in a big rowing motion. Bring them up toward the ears then squeeze them together in front of your chest. Then let them drop. Finally, pull your shoulders back and try to touch your shoulder blades together. Do the entire cycle three times. Then reverse the cycle three more times. You can repeat this whole sequence throughout the day as often as you like.

Lower Back ● "Most, but not all, lower back problems involve muscle tightness, weakness, and spasm," says Dr. Nagler. No wonder—we subject this vulnerable region to all kinds of stress. "The lumbar spine is the 'abused link' in the body," says Zeb Kendrick, Ph.D., director of the biokinetics research laboratory at Temple University. Lower-back tension and aches may be symptoms of imbalance elsewhere. "Back pain may occur because of problems with the ankles, knees, hips, and shoulders," he says. Postural analysis by a physical therapist could help pinpoint a "structural" problem. High heels are a possible source of lower-back pain, as they can throw the body out of alignment.

Improper use of the body plus weak or tense muscles adds up to a potential for trouble in the lower back. The problem can range from a minor injury or strain to a full-blown muscle spasm. The cause is usually easy to identify. Maybe you lifted a heavy box or lunged awkwardly to catch a falling object in midair. "Any bending, reaching, or twisting that takes the back beyond its protective limits can strain the ligaments," says Dr. Resnick. When the back "goes out," that usually means that a muscle spasm has resulted in pressure on the nerve, says Dr. Fahrion.

Relief: For mild tension in the lower back, try this exercise: Lie on your back, knees bent, feet flat, and arms by your sides. Slowly roll up as far as you can. Hold for a count of three and roll back down. Then bring your knees up toward your nose, hold for a count of three and lower feet to floor. Do five cycles twice a day. Switching to flats or low-heeled shoes may also bring some relief.

Severe back pain should always be evaluated by a doctor. For muscle spasms, he or she will probably prescribe rest, pain-relieving medications and ice massage followed by heat. "The best and easiest way to relieve muscle spasm is simply to rest and immobilize the part that's injured," says Dr. Resnick. (Pills advertised for lower-back spasm are analgesics, not muscle relaxants, he notes.) Finally, the muscles simply need some time to recover. "The vast majority of lower-back strains heal by about four weeks," he says.

Prevention: Treat your back with respect. When you lift, bend your knees and use your leg muscles, not your back, for strength. Carry objects close to your body. To ease your back as you sit, Dr. Kendrick suggests making a "lumbar roll": Roll up a small towel and place it horizontally in the small of your back. Lean against it, being careful to maintain an upright posture. Regular walking or other gentle exercise can also abolish chronic low back pain.

Medical Help for the "Thin-Skinned"

Does your skin chap in cold winds, crack from dry heat, "crawl" in woolen turtlenecks or react to certain salves, scents, cleaning solutions, or even the rubber gloves you wear to protect your hands from harsh detergents? If so, you probably know from experience what to avoid. But do you know how to "condition" your skin to resist irritation in the first place?

"Preventing skin irritations really requires a two-pronged effort," says Richard Odom, M.D., professor of dermatology at the University of California in San Francisco and president of the American Academy of Dermatology. "First, identify the substance you're sensitive to and avoid contact. And second, take care to maintain the integrity of your skin's natural barrier cover. Skin that's healthy and intact is better able to resist irritations, allergic reactions, even bacterial and fungal infections."

Actually, the skin is designed for the purpose of protection. Its armor of keratin (the same protein component of nails and hair) shields it from irritants, allergens and a multitude of microorganisms. Its cellular renewal system, which continually replaces old surface cells with new, discourages colonization by bacteria and fungi. And, in the event of a solar assault, its production of extra pigment (melanin) offers some protection against the damaging effects of ultraviolet light.

Unfortunately, the system is not fail-safe.

Who's Vulnerable?

"For any person—or group of people—the effectiveness of the skin's protective barrier varies tremendously," says Dr. Odom. The thin skin of the eyelids, scrotum, and labia is especially susceptible to penetration by irritants and allergens—as are sun-damaged areas, which tend to be drier and thinner than normal skin. The underarms, groin, and toe webs are vulnerable sites for bacterial and fungal infections.

Then, too, some people are inherently more sensitive than others. Fair skin and a history of hay fever, asthma and eczema (weeping skin irritations) identify the extremely vulnerable type. "These people tend to have dry skin that itches incessantly, especially at the bends of the elbows and behind the knees, and is easily irritated by heat, cold, and a wide variety of cosmetic agents," Dr. Odom explains.

But even "normal" skin can be sensitive sometimes. "To some extent, it's a matter of exposure," says Robert M. Adams, M.D., clinical professor of dermatology at Stanford University

Medical Center. "The fact is, under certain conditions, anything can irritate the skin—even water, if it's too hot or too cold or used excessively."

Likewise, allergic-type skin reactions can strike just about anyone at any time. "We are not born allergic to nickel, rubber, poison ivy, or any other contact allergen," says Dr. Adams. "We develop sensitivities during the course of our life's activities."

New products and new avenues of exposure may be the reason dermatologists are treating more skin-sensitivity problems than ever before. The fitness arena, for example, is proving to be fertile ground for irritations.

With the growing popularity of hot tubs and fitness clubs, athlete's foot and other fungal, yeast, and bacterial infections are on the rise. Rodney Basler, M.D., consultant in dermatology to the University of Nebraska, Lincoln, and director of the American Academy of Dermatology's forum on sports medicine, also reports an increase in the number of cases of allergic contact dermatitis caused by the rubber in shoes, swimming goggles, and waistbands on athletic clothes. "Depending too on when, where, and how hard you work out, sun, wind, heat, and perspiration can exacerbate sensitive-skin problems," he says.

Reducing Water Damage

Moisture can undermine the skin's protective barrier. This is especially true in warm, occluded areas, particularly the toes and groin, where perspiration may accumulate. "Perspiration softens the outer layer of skin and in so doing, decreases the barrier effect," explains Dr. Basler. "This allows penetration by yeast, bacteria, and fungi, which tend to thrive in the warm, moist environment."

Heat and perspiration also sensitize the skin to irritations from wool, certain chemicals in synthetic fibers (most notably formaldehyde), and detergent residue leached from clothing by sweat. Another reason to keep supersensitive skin cool: Perspiration can aggravate existing problems, such as eczema in the elbow crease.

To reduce skin damage from perspiration accumulation, dermatologists recommend the following steps.

● Put on socks and underwear when skin is dry, not damp. To speed drying in moisture-sensitive areas, such as the underarms, groin, and toes, blow the skin dry with a hair dryer—cool setting, please.

● Wear lightweight, loose-fitting clothes made of "breathable" fabrics—even in the wintertime. Heavy clothes occlude perspiration. Plus, bacteria and fungi find excellent breeding grounds in the warm, damp skin under winter clothing. Layer for warmth, with nonirritating fabrics closest to skin.

● If you're planning an activity that involves heavy sweating, wear absorbent clothes, such as cotton T-shirts and sweats. Long-sleeved cotton T-shirts help prevent perspiration irritations of existing elbow eczema. Change into dry clothes as soon as possible after exercise.

● Launder synthetic clothes and workout wear two or three times before wearing. This will remove potential irritants that otherwise may be leached out of the fabrics by perspiration.

● For active outdoor winter activities, wrap a cotton terrycloth towel around your neck rather than a woolen scarf. This nonirritating material will protect you from the drying winter winds and absorb excess perspiration.

● If you are prone to perspire in heavy socks and boots, dust your feet with a talc-free powder or spray them with an antiperspirant. Although cornstarch is frequently used as a substitute for powder, its nutrient effect may actually promote microbial growth in some cases, says Dr. Basler. *Note:* Do not apply powder or spray to irritated or broken skin or if you know that you are sensitive to antiperspirants.

Dealing with Dryness Damage

While sweat accumulation is a major threat to certain skin areas, the exact opposite—extreme dryness—can weaken the skin's barrier too.

Dryness is the catch-22 of sensitive skin: Skin that's irritated (from heat, cold, wind, sun, soap, or water) becomes dry. And, conversely, dry skin is easily irritated.

Leonard Swinyer, M.D., associate clinical professor of medicine in the Division of Dermatology at the University of Utah Health Science Center in Salt Lake City, explains. "Think of the surface of your skin as a tiled roof," he says. "Like roofing shingles, overlapping skin cells form a barrier against outside elements. However, when skin cells (which consist of about 65 percent water) dry out, they shrink. The cell 'shingles' separate from one another, resulting in a leaky roof easily penetrable by outside irritants."

The drier the skin, the greater the damage to the barrier cover. "If the skin is so dry it splits or cracks, the problem is compounded," he adds. "Anything you apply to broken skin— even a moisturizing lotion—can seep through the cracks and possibly irritate the underside of the skin."

Dry, damaged skin invites allergic reactions as well. "Allergens penetrate better when the skin has been broken or injured," says Dr. Adams. "A person's skin may react to a weak allergen in a cream, for example, only when the product is applied to chapped or irritated skin. When the skin is intact, the same product produces no allergic reaction. Similarly, a person with chapped hands may wear rubber gloves to protect the skin from further irritation—then wind up reacting to chemicals in the rubber."

Apparently, too, the skin does not have to be extensively damaged to qualify as a site for the development of allergic contact dermatitis. "Minor inflamed patches of dryness and irritation the size of a quarter or half dollar will do," says William Jordan, M.D., professor of dermatology at the Medical College of Virginia, Richmond.

No one knows the exact mechanism that causes skin to dry out. But the latest theory is that it has to do with moisture-retaining compounds on the skin's surface. "People with sensitive skin who are especially prone to dryness may have a lower concentration of these natural moisturizing factors. Or these factors may not function as well in some people as in others," says Dr. Swinyer.

"In any case, all dryness is due either to an inherent inability of the skin to hold on to water or to the evaporation of water off the skin," he adds. "Here in Utah both factors contribute to the problem. Not only do we have a large number of residents with inherently dry, sensitive skin, but we also have very low humidity, which accelerates evaporation."

To some extent, sebum (oil), which floats over the surface of skin, retards moisture loss. If you don't have oily skin, you can create the same effect with moisturizing creams or lotions. But Dr. Swinyer contends that the key to preventing dry skin is not so much in retaining or creating an oily moisture barrier but in preserving the skin's own natural moisturizing factors.

Soap and water remove these moisturizing compounds from the skin. With excessive use, the skin's barrier becomes irritated and the loss of these moisturizing factors accelerates. Temporarily, then, the skin cannot hang on to water.

Fortunately, new moisturizing factors are continually produced at a deeper skin level. But, as Dr. Swinyer points out, it takes about 30 days for them to reach the surface. And if underlying cells have been injured any time in their passage to the surface, then they will not be prepared to hold on to water once they get to the top.

To determine just how dry your skin is, Dr. Swinyer recommends this simple test: Put a strip of Scotch tape on your arm or leg (the face is generally too oily for this test). Pull it off and transfer the tape to black construction paper. Viewing the tape on the paper, you will see a pattern of skin cells. The more the cells clump together, the drier the skin. If the cells appear evenly distributed, the skin has adequate moisture.

Preventing Dry-Skin Problems

To prevent skin damage from moisture evaporation, dermatologists recommend the following measures.

● Keep your house on the cool side. Not only will this reduce perspiration under bulky winter clothes, it will increase the humidity content of the air.

● Apply a creamy sunscreen before extended winter outings to ski, skate, or walk. Not only will this prevent moisture evaporation from the wind and cold, it will protect you against the drying effect of ultraviolet light.

● Postpone shaving or washing exposed areas in the morning before facing the elements. The natural sebum offers some protection from the wind and cold.

● Use soap sparingly. Be sure to rinse.

● Avoid long, leisurely baths or showers and stay out of hot water (including hot tubs). "The longer you stay in water, the more you soak away the natural moisturizing factors," says Dr. Swinyer. He recommends quick, cool showers.

● Avoid steam baths and saunas. Excessive sweating can float the moisturizing factor off and dry your skin. From that standpoint, there's no advantage in the moist heat of a steam bath over the dry heat of a sauna.

● Apply moisturizers to damp — not dry — skin. A moisturizer simply seals in moisture. If you apply it to dry skin, the skin underneath stays dry.

● To cleanse the face of dirt and excess oil (without drying it out), Dr. Swinyer recommends using a mild cleansing lotion designed for sensitive skin or a lipid-free moisturizing/cleansing lotion, such as Cetaphil (available at pharmacies). Apply the lotion to the skin with your fingers, and pat it off with a soft cotton towel (don't rinse it off and don't use tissues). Then, while the skin is still damp, apply a moisturizer. Avoid astringents, which remove moisture with the oils.

● While it's important to protect chapped or irritated hands from hot water or detergents, the allergy-prone should wear cotton gloves underneath their rubber ones.

Heel-to-Toe Foot-Care Tips

Attractive feet are soft, smooth, supple, and especially, healthy. Keeping them that way takes special care. But, first, you've got to undo any signs of neglect, such as dry, cracked skin, corns, and calluses.

"If you have any fissures that have developed a bacterial infection, get those taken care of by a podiatrist before you start your own foot-care program," says podiatrist Terry L. Spilken, D.P.M., whose work with athletic and dance groups, including the Alvin Ailey American Dance Theatre, allows him to see more than his share of foot problems.

"If you have corns, you may find temporary relief by using flannel pads that fit around them," he says. "Just switching to more comfortable shoes can sometimes resolve the problem. If it doesn't, you'll need medical help."

Calluses can usually be handled at home. But be patient. Attacking callused skin too aggressively can irritate it and do more harm than good. "Use a pumice stone or Buf Puf to remove a few layers of callused skin each night," says Dr. Spilken. "Never use a razor blade on calluses because of the risk of infection."

Pampering Your Feet

For foot models Karen Williamson and Nina Reeves, both of the Ford Modeling Agency, healthy, good-looking feet are their fortune. "I can't afford to let my feet go, so I see a podiatrist every two or three weeks," Williamson explains. "In between I keep my feet pumiced and as callus-free as possible." Williamson, Reeves, and Dr. Spilken offer these tips on foot care.

● Have a professional pedicure. This gives you a good basis on which to begin your own foot-care program.
● Spend five minutes in the tub before you pumice your feet. This allows your skin time to soften. Then use a moisturizing cream with the pumice stone to gently scour away dried skin.
● Groom your nails after you shower or bathe. The warm water softens nails and cuticles so they're easier to cut and shape.
● Using an emery board, file nails in one direction only. If you have weak or fragile nails, use the finer side of the emery board.
● Toe cuticles usually don't require special care. If they get high, gently file them with an emery board. Don't cut them. If you're too aggressive in grooming them, you may find that they need your attention more often.
● To clean cuticles, use a soft nail brush or an old toothbrush.
● Nail polish is fine for healthy toenails. If you have a nail that is discolored, thick, painful, or pulling away from the nail bed, avoid polishing it. There may be an underlying fungus or yeast infection, which should be treated by your podiatrist.

● To remove old nail polish, use nonacetone polish remover. It won't dry out your toenails.

● Dry your feet thoroughly with a blow dryer set on low. Be certain to dry the area between your toes. Then apply dusting powder to absorb perspiration and moisture. If you have sensitive skin, choose a powder that's fragrance-free. If you have athlete's foot, look for one with fungus-fighting ingredients.

● Moisturize feet daily. After a few weeks, you may be able to reduce this treatment to once a week and still remain callus-free. If at any time a callus becomes painful, see a podiatrist.

● Apply a rich moisturizing cream to your feet at night. For added effect, wear socks to bed.

Shoe Savvy

Don't ruin all your foot-care efforts by wearing the wrong shoes. "If a certain pair of shoes hurts your feet, get rid of them. Shoes can actually change the shape of your toes," says Williamson.

To prevent corns and calluses, wear shoes that fit properly, that give support and protection without reshaping your foot. The shoe should be roomy enough to allow a forefinger's width between the shoe's tip and your longest toe, but not so loose that your foot slides around. The widest part of your foot should correspond to the widest part of the shoe. Never buy a shoe that's not comfortable in the store on the theory that it will stretch out as you wear it. And never buy shoes if you can see the side of the shoe is stretched out by your foot.

A tip from Dr. Spilken: The best time to try on shoes is late afternoon, when your feet are more likely to be slightly swollen.

To help keep your feet supple, Dr. Spilken suggests these exercises.

1. Curl your toes in and hold to a count of five. Then slowly release and flex your foot. Switch feet and repeat five times.

2. Sit with your toes on the ground and your heels off. Press into the floor and release. Repeat five times.

3. Sit with your heels together. Put a towel on the floor at your right foot and try to move it to between your feet by pushing with the front part of your feet and keeping your heels together. Put the towel at your left side and repeat.

4. Try to actually pick up the towel with your toes using one foot at a time. Repeat five times.

A Foot Note: Massage

For tired aching feet, massage can be just what the doctor ordered. Try it after your bath or shower. Rest your left foot on your right knee. Then, using the heel of your hand, massage your foot in a circular motion. Work from one end of your foot to the other. For more direct force, go back and knead the arch with your thumbs. Move along the sole and sides of your foot. Flex each toe back individually and gently rotate it. Tug it gently. Switch feet and repeat.

The Healing Art of Self-Massage

Whack! You smack your funny bone. Oowwww! A sudden cramp clenches your calf. Ooohh! You awake with a stiff neck.

What's the very first thing you do (after you let out a good yelp)? You reach out to rub where it hurts. And for good reason: Rubbing works. In fact, doctors and scientists are discovering that there may be more pain-easing power in a good rub than you realize.

One explanation of how rubbing dampens pain is called the "gate control theory," says Edward Resnick, M.D., professor of orthopedic surgery and director of the Pain Control Center at Temple University Hospital. "Pain impulses run toward the spinal cord and then up the cord and into the brain," he says. "It's only when they reach the brain that these impulses are perceived as pain. Rubbing can send other impulses along the same nerves and interfere with the pain impulses. In this way, rubbing can 'close the gate' that pain impulses have to pass through."

Rules of the Rub

However it works, rubbing is proving to be serious medicine for a whole lot of hurts. Here's what some experts can teach us about using rub power against everyday aches and pains.

Temperature Control ● "For your basic aches and pains, use heat first," says Phil Dunphy, a registered physical therapist and exercise physiologist who runs the HEAR (Health through Exercise and Rehabilitation) Institute in New Jersey. He and other experts believe that you can get the most from a rub or massage by first warming up the affected muscle.

"Moist heat is best," explains Brad Green, D.O., attending orthopedic surgeon at Sturdy Memorial Hospital in Attleboro, Massachusetts. "You can use either a warm shower or one of those hydro-collator packs that you boil in water and then wrap in a towel. They really send off waves of moist heat. They're especially good for back problems."

Self-Massage ● Try giving yourself a massage (the ultimate rub!) on the muscles that hurt. It's easy. You just have to keep a few pointers in mind.

First, when you rub, gently move the skin over the underlying tissue, using a circular motion. Then occasionally rub toward the heart in long sweeps and try direct pressure on the muscles. Use your fingertips, thumbs, knuckles—whatever it takes.

"But don't be rough," says Dunphy. "People always go too fast and try to do too much too soon. Be gentle. Maybe go back and work on the area two or three times during the day instead of trying to do it all at once."

And rub smart. Don't use massage on a serious injury or inflamed area. Don't use it if you have phlebitis or other vascular problems. And don't continue massaging if the pain increases. When in doubt, seek out a licensed massage therapist.

Ice Treatment ● While heat can prepare the body for rubbing, cooling the painful area with ice while you massage can enhance the benefits, says the originator of the gate control theory, Ronald Melzack, Ph.D., past president of the International Association for the Study of Pain.

"There's a large and convincing body of literature on the use of cold to relieve aches and pains," he says. "The intense stimulation that ice provides is an excellent way to 'close the gate' at the spinal pathway and inhibit painful information from reaching your brain. The basic technique [for ice massage] is to slowly rub the ice in circles on the spot that hurts. Do it for five to seven minutes or until the area feels numb."

You can use an ice cube, he says, or a bag of frozen peas for large areas.

Higher Altitude ● For leg muscles, let gravity help you, says Ed Moore, the massage therapist who rubbed away the aches and pains of the 1984 U.S. Olympic cycling team. "Elevate the area you're rubbing," he says, "so gravity works with you to stimulate the blood flow."

Special Rubs for Special Hurts

All pain is not created equal. So here's the experts' list of rubs customized for specific sore spots.

Dental Pain ● To ease an achy tooth, you rub what? Your tooth? No, researchers say, you rub your hand.

"We've shown," says Dr. Melzack, "that you can relieve intense dental pain by 50 percent or more simply by rubbing an ice cube into the V-shaped area where the bones of the thumb and forefinger meet (not the web). All you have to do is rub the ice gently over the area for five to seven minutes. Don't rub for longer than that."

In a series of experiments, Dr. Melzack reports, ice massage eased dental pain in 60 to 90 percent of the people who tried it. Later research indicated that the technique worked with either hand, not just the one on the side of the dental pain.

Charley Horse ● This pain in the calf, says Dr. Green, is a muscle spasm. "The calf muscle can cramp up so badly that it will actually point your foot toward the floor."

Dr. Green's prescription for rubbing: Pull your toes back toward you while gently rubbing your calf. Start behind the knee and slide your hand down the muscle to the heel, then repeat. Always rub with the muscle, not across it.

Neck Pain ● For run-of-the-mill sore neck muscles, first hit the showers. Direct a warm spray on the sore spot. Then gently rub the area with your three middle fingers, moving them in small circles.

For a stiff neck, Dr. Melzack says ice massage works well. Use your fingers to find the sensitive spot on the neck and shoulder area, then rub ice on it.

Sinus Headache ● "A steady rubbing pressure on certain areas of the face may open up the sinuses and relieve the congestion that's causing the headache," Dr. Green says. "Rub around the ridge of bone located just above and below your eyes. You can also rub your cheeks directly in line with those points, just above your teeth."

Sore Hands ● To beat the soreness, try whole-hand massage. Start by slowly opening and closing them. Then rub the palms in a circular motion. Keep fingers together while squeezing and pressing them. Spread them, then gently squeeze and pull each one. Then, using a lubricant (any vegetable oil or mois- turizing lotion will do), rub from wrist to fingertips and back again. Do this repeatedly, rubbing both sides of the hand. Then stroke the forearm, rubbing toward the elbow and back, squeezing the muscles like a sponge.

Ed Moore says that hand massage works best if your hand is resting on a firm surface, such as a tabletop, for support. "You can really use your body weight then," he explains.

Backache ● For low back pain, consider an ice rub where it smarts. And for pain where you can't reach, try—would you believe?—tennis balls. They're Moore's unorthodox solution to the problem of self-massage for the back. "You get two tennis balls," explains Moore, "and lie down so they slide under the small of your back, one on each side of your spine.

Take a deep breath, relax and slowly work them up your back. You can vary the pressure by simply shifting your weight around.

"You can 'rub' your whole back in ten minutes or spend ten minutes just in one problem area. If you place the sole of your foot on the opposite knee (let the knee fall to the outside) and slide tennis balls under your hip, you can massage your hip area as well. Just remember to do some gentle stretching exercises first—like raising your arms toward the ceiling and back down again."

The Practical Psychology of Positive Living

Think It; Heal It!

A new understanding of why some people get sick when exposed to germs while others remain healthy is radically revising the popular concept of what causes illness.

Recent research has demonstrated, for instance, how our immunity is affected by what goes on in our heads, by hormonal changes resulting from poor coping, or by direct effects of our central nervous system.

Our cognitions (thoughts, beliefs, attitudes) and the social support we perceive in our lives can alter the levels of our hormones and neurotransmitters, the chemical messengers that carry on communication between our cells and that largely govern the activity of many of our physical processes. Excessive stress hormones like cortisol and catecholamines, for example, can lead to artery damage, cholesterol buildup, and heart disease. As we will see, chronic high levels of these chemicals can diminish the activity of antibodies and natural killer cells that protect us against foreign invaders and tumors. Deficient suppressor cells may permit overreaction of the immune system to the point that the body starts attacking itself, as in rheumatoid arthritis.

The Mind/Body Meld

The connections between mental and bodily processes are real and anatomical. To say "it's only in your head" or "it's just your imagination" as a way of dismissing pain or illness is

186

to deny physical fact. The hypothalamus control center of the brain, for instance, is directly "wired" to the immune system. If a portion of the hypothalamus is electrically stimulated, antibodies increase. If it is cut, immune activity is depressed.

Thoughts, beliefs, and imagination are not ephemeral abstractions but electrochemical events with physiological consequences. Sophisticated instrumentation such as PET scanning now permits us to see the brain in action as thinking occurs and to map blood flow in the cerebral hemispheres as thoughts and feelings change. Advances in radioimmunoassay techniques make it possible to pick up hormonal changes as a function of different appraisals of stressful situations.

Recent findings have repeatedly affirmed the link between mind and health. A sense of control can keep our stress chemicals from reaching damaging levels while we are under pressure. An openness to change and an attitude of involvement can increase our resistance to illness.

On the other hand, a sense of helplessness can depress our immune system and decrease our resistance. A belief that we must have power and dominance can also affect our immunity when we are under stress. A giving-up reaction to life stresses can increase our risk of sudden death or cancer. A chronically hostile, cynical, or distrusting attitude can contribute to our risk of atherosclerosis and heart disease.

"Proof" of the mind's influence on the body has grown rapidly in the last few decades. But as recently as the 1950s, skeptics were arguing that there were no nerves connecting the brain to our anterior pituitary (the body's "master gland"), and thus there was no way a stressful thought or appraisal could trigger release of powerful stress hormones. The connection was confirmed, however, when it was shown that a rich network of blood vessels links the brain's hypothalamus to the pituitary. Simple brain peptides—small molecules of amino acids—travel down the vessels and stimulate the pituitary, which in turn activates release of adrenal cortical hormones.

In 1977, Roger Guillemin and Andrew Schally received the Nobel Prize after demonstrating how the brain uses these chemical messengers to "give orders" to the body. Working independently, these two scientists isolated a series of tiny molecules that are made in the brain's hypothalamus and travel to the pituitary, where they then affect the functioning of our thyroids, adrenals, gonads, and the very course of our growth.

Immunologists have suspected for years that stress hormones affect people's immunity. Robert Good, former president and director of Memorial Sloan-Kettering Cancer Hospital in New York, was one of the first authorities in the field to recognize that "a positive attitude" and "a constructive frame of mind," as well as depression, may alter our ability to resist "infections, allergies, autoimmunities, or even cancer."

Just how our reactions to stress and our ability to cope affect our resistance to disease is the focus of intensive research. Much remains to be clarified, but it is known that the immune system is directly influenced by nerve impulses from the brain as well as by hormones that are increased by stress reactions.

Another important bodily system affected by how we view life and react to stressful situations is the heart and our arteries. People who are cynical or have hostile attitudes or suppressed anger have been found to have more atherosclerosis and blockage of coronary arteries. And they are more likely to experience heart attacks.

Individuals who are in a chronic struggle to exert domination and control—Type-A personalites—may also be "coronary prone," particularly if they are hostile. Chronic activation of the fight-or-flight response means that the neurotransmitter norepinephrine is liberated in increased amounts from the ends of sympathetic-nervous-system fibers, acting upon blood vessels, the heart, and other organs. Excessive norepinephrine has also been associated with hostile attitudes. In excessive amounts it may do damage to the lining of coronary arteries, provide a chemical insult to the heart muscle, promote high blood pressure, and disturb platelets and red blood cells—all of which can contribute to the increased risk of a myocardial infarction or some other form of serious heart disease. The constant turning on of fight-or-flight responses can also trigger a coronary artery spasm, which may result in a heart attack.

Overreactions to stress may stir up other biochemical changes that can threaten our cardiac health. Cholesterol levels rise and uric acid goes up[$^{}$], and each of these has been associated with coronary heart disease.

The Power of Feeling Close

When social contact is increased or loneliness reduced, the immune system seems to strengthen. A group of 30 elderly people in retirement homes showed increased immune competence in terms of both natural killer (NK) cells and antibodies from being visited three times a week for a month. Support can also affect T-cells (which control and coordinate the immune system) when a person is under stress. Lack of support has been found to reduce suppressor T-cells and is associated with recurrence of some illnesses such as herpes simplex type 2.

In women, the immune system seems to be sensitive to the social support that comes from a good marriage. In a study of 38 married women, researchers at Ohio State University College of Medicine found that marital quality was significantly associated with immune functioning, including percent of helper T-cells and ratio of helper to suppressor lymphocytes. The women who perceived their marriages as satisfying and supportive had less depression and loneliness as well as better immune defenses.

Having frank and confiding relationships may be a critical element in whether social support protects our health. In other words, it may be more important to have at least one person with whom we can share open and honest thoughts and feelings than it is to have a whole network of more superficial relationships. Researchers at the University of New Mexico School of Medicine found that, among 256 healthy elderly people, individuals with confiding relationships had significantly higher indices of immune function, and lower serum cholesterol and uric-acid levels.

Bad Feelings, Bad Infections

Type 2 herpes, which is venereal herpes, has been found to recur when people with the latent virus anticipate stressful events ahead, experience negative moods, or lack social support. A study at the University of California School of Medicine in

San Francisco showed that both helper and suppressor T-cells are affected by perceptions of stress and by negative moods.

Psychologist Margaret Kemeny and her coworkers found among 36 people with genital herpes that those who were depressed experienced more recurrences of symptoms. The depressed individuals also had significantly lower levels of suppressor cytotoxic T-cells, which apparently keep outbreaks from occurring. Depression, stress, anxiety, hostility, fatigue — all were found to be significant predictors of poor functioning of suppressor T-cells.

Latent bacteria as well as viruses may be activated by negative moods and distress. For instance, bacteria normally residing in the mouth may produce trench-mouth sores, technically called acute necrotizing ulcerative gingivitis (ANUG). People who become stressed before examinations and have depression of their IgA antibodies, which are a first-line defense against infection, have been found to get trench-mouth sores.

Even the bacteria in our mouths that contribute to dental caries have been found to increase when we perceive situations as stressful. When we relax, amounts of such salivary bacteria decline.

A Prescription for Stronger Immunity

The importance of relaxation in keeping the immune system strong has been demonstrated by psychologist Janice Kiecolt-Glaser and her research group at Ohio State. They found that medical students had decreases in helper T-cells on the day of examinations. But when half the group was taught relaxation exercises, their T-cells increased. The percentage of their helper T-cells could be predicted by how frequently the students practiced relaxation. The researchers suggest that these data provide further evidence that relaxation may be able to enhance at least some component of cellular immunity, and thus might ultimately be useful in influencing the incidence and course of disease.

Other studies have shown that stress hormones, such as cortisol and the catecholamines, decrease after relaxation. Because our immune defenses tend to weaken when we generate stress hormones, relaxation exercises may be one way to keep our resistance up.

Love Takes Health a Step Further

When we tone down our negative thoughts and beliefs, we seem to be less susceptible to illness. But being less negative is one thing, being positive another. We have more evidence on the negative, but at last some scientific attention is being given to the positive as it affects our health.

Just as we know there is such a thing as "mind-made disease"—illness largely triggered by our own stressful thoughts and behaviors—there is good reason to believe that "mind-made health" is also a reality.

Psychologist David McClelland of Harvard has found that when students were shown a film designed to inspire feelings of love and caring, an antibody—salivary IgA—increased, providing major protection against colds and upper-respiratory infection. The film they saw was on Mother Teresa, the nun who won a Nobel peace prize for her work in caring for the poor on the streets of Calcutta.

Even those who professed intense dislike for Mother Teresa— some said she was a fake and that her work did no good— showed immune function improvement. Such a finding is consistent with McClelland's theory that deeper, unconscious beliefs and motives determine people's bodily reactions and their behavior more than do conscious cognitions. He thinks a figure like Mother Teresa reaches "the consciously disapproving people in a part of their brains that they are unaware of and that is still responding to the strength of her tender loving care."

When the students were shown a film on Attila the Hun, their antibody levels dropped. Salivary IgA levels also decrease when people see a film that evokes feelings of helplessness, which suggests why a sense of control can help protect health.

Having as a trait the ability to love and care about others seems to result in lower levels of the stress hormone norepinephrine and a higher ratio of helper/suppressor T-cells, an important balance in a healthy immune system. Less illness is associated with the caring trait.

McClelland has also tested for the physiological effects of intimacy. People with high scores on intimacy have higher levels of IgA antibodies and report less serious illness. In addition, he has found that people who seek friendship and affiliation with others are generally more healthy.

In Topeka, Kansas, at the Menninger Clinic, tests showed that people who are romantically in love suffer fewer colds and have white blood cells that more actively fight infection. The lovers are also reported to have lower levels of lactic acid in their blood, which means they are less likely to get tired, and higher levels of endorphins, which may contribute to a sense of euphoria and may reduce pain.

McClelland acknowledges that "we don't have any idea about how love aids the lymphocytes and improves immune functions," but the evidence strongly suggests it does.

Bernard Siegel, an assistant clinical professor of surgery at Yale Medical School who has been a practicing surgeon for more than 30 years, predicts that "someday we will understand the physiological and psychological workings of love well enough to turn on its full force more reliably. Once it is scientific, it will be accepted."

Other evidence also suggests that caring is a potent mediator of bodily responses. Persons who have pets to care for have been found to recover faster from illnesses. People with myocardial infarctions who own animals have been reported to have one-half the mortality rate of those who do not have pets.

Among patients in hospitals who have had heart attacks, those with pets waiting for them live longer after returning home. Pets also seem to help us be more optimistic, another quality that contributes to better health.

Giving people something to care for can enhance their sense of control in life. When a group of nursing home residents was given plants of their own to take care of and was urged to assume more responsibility for themselves as well, they reported a greater sense of control and showed significant improvement in their health and activity. They also lived longer.

The effects of tender loving care on both animals and humans can be profound. Rabbits on a high-fat diet that were talked to and petted developed significantly less atherosclerosis than those that received only routine treatment in the laboratory. Women surgical patients whose hands were held by a nurse while blood pressure and temperature were taken were able to leave the hospital sooner and recovered faster when they got home.

Beauty and the Body

A number of years ago, psychologist Abraham Maslow, in proposing that a hierarchy of needs motivates human behavior, suggested that beauty promotes health. When we are moved by music, the beauty of nature, or a work of art, we apparently "turn on" and release in the brain opioid substances—endorphins or similar peptides—that give us goose bumps, "thrills" or other sensations of pleasure.

Various studies have shown that nature scenes—views of water and vegetation, particularly—elicit positive feelings in people, reduce anxiety in those who are stressed, and significantly increase the amplitude of alpha brain waves. High alpha amplitude is associated with feelings of relaxation. When we experience beauty, then, we seem less likely to have stressful thoughts and physiological arousal.

Roger Ulrich, in the Department of Geography at the University of Delaware, tested the effects of hospital room views on the recovery of patients who had undergone gallbladder surgery. Twenty-three patients were in rooms that overlooked a stand of trees with foliage. A matched group of 23 other patients who had gallbladder surgery in the same hospital had a view of a brick wall from their rooms. Those with the tree view spent significantly less time in the hospital after surgery, required substantially less painkilling medication, and had fewer negative ratings from nurses on their recovery.

The Health Power of Hope

Research on people who live longer shows that they characteristically have a sense of hope, order, and control in their lives. "The hope habit" seems to encourage longevity by reducing the effects of stress on the body and turning on self-healing systems.

Shlomo Breznitz, a researcher from the University of

Haifa in Israel, who is at the National Institute of Mental Health studying hope, is convinced that hopeful patterns of thinking can be cultivated like any habit of discipline—brushing our teeth, for instance. Thinking hopefully is the opposite of being a doomsayer or fatalist. Someone with the hope habit whose father died at 55 will say, "I'm going to live my life so I'll beat those odds," rather than, "My father died at 55, so I guess no matter what I do, I will, too."

Another hope researcher, psychiatrist Louis A. Gottschalk of the University of California at Irvine, believes that spiritual faith helps people lead more hopeful and less stressful lives. Gottschalk and his coworkers developed a way to measure how much hope people have by doing a content analysis of samples of their speech. They found that among 16 patients with various metastatic cancers, those with higher hope scores prior to treatment survived significantly longer. A substantial correlation also was found between hope and survival in a group of 27 cancer patients undergoing radiation therapy at Cincinnati General Hospital.

The Optimist's Edge

Although our outlook clearly affects the degree of stress we feel and our physiological reactions, the effects of being optimistic have only recently been researched. Psychologists Michael Scheier of Carnegie-Mellon University, in Pittsburgh, and Charles Carver of the University of Miami found that optimism was a predictor of physical well-being. Among some 140 undergraduates under the stress of deadlines and impending exams, those who were more optimistic reported being less bothered by physical symptoms than did the students who were inclined to be pessimistic.

The psychologists decided that the optimistic students coped more effectively with problems and were thus less likely to experience physical symptoms of any magnitude from stress.

In addition, an optimistic outlook may, in itself, activate protective healing systems.

Other research has indicated that an optimistic attitude is also a key factor in living longer and getting sick less often. People who are optimistic about their own health, for instance, have been shown to be at reduced risk of dying. This is true even if "objective" measures—laboratory tests, doctor examinations—show them to be in poor health. In contrast, people who believe they are in poor health but objectively are in good or excellent health have an increased mortality risk.

Such findings were documented in a study of 3,128 people 65 years and older in Manitoba, Canada. They were surveyed in 1971, and records were gathered from physicians and hospitals on their health status. The Canadians, none of whom were in institutions, were then tracked for the next six years. Even when differences in age, sex, income, residence, and life satisfaction were controlled for, those who believed their health was excellent had one-third the risk of death of those who perceived that their health was poor.

In the United States, even more dramatic findings came from the Alameda County, California, study of 6,928 adults, whose health was kept track of for nine years. The mortality risk for the "health pessimists" among men was some two times greater than that for the "health optimists," and the mortality risk was a striking five times greater among women.

Although nobody knows for sure exactly how optimistic or pessimistic beliefs about the state of one's health may influence chances of dying, there is the possibility that such perceptions affect our resistance to disease. We have seen that through the central nervous system, beliefs and attitudes can affect the immune system and affect our susceptibility to illness. A sense of optimism and control seems to protect against both impairment of immune defenses and damage to the cardiovascular system.

The Happiness Factor

The interdependence of happiness and health has been demonstrated in several long-term studies. In a study of 268 volunteers that controlled for the effects of age, work satisfaction and happiness were found to predict longevity better than any health or physical activity factor. A significant association between perceptions of life satisfaction and health was also reported among different groups of men and women whose illnesses were charted over 20 years.

The quality of a person's marriage, as he or she perceives it, has been found to be a more powerful predictor of happiness than even satisfaction with work or relationships with friends. Marital satisfaction is significantly associated with both level of immune functioning and psychological well-being. A prospective study of 10,000 men in Israel showed that their risk of developing angina pectoris was nearly two times lower if they answered yes to the question "Does your wife show you her love?"

Humor as Medicine

One study reports that finding something funny results in a significant increase in IgA antibodies. People who customarily use humor as a coping method have been found to have higher concentrations of these antibodies.

Pleasant moods, such as mirthful ones, are associated with changes in levels of stress hormones, such as epinephrine and norepinephrine.

In a study by the Laughter Project at the University of California at Santa Barbara, researchers found that laughter was as effective as biofeedback training in reducing stress. And, they said, one advantage laughter has as a stress reducer is that it "requires no special training, no special equipment, and no special laboratory. All it requires is a funny bone."

The "Vitamin" for Heart and Soul

Much of what social scientists know about friendships, families, and marriages ought to be stamped: "Made in Japan."

That's where researchers have found that there is more to a happy, fulfilling relationship than whether it makes you feel all warm and mushy inside. It might also keep you *healthy* inside.

In many ways, the Japanese have much in common with those of us here in the West: cigarette smoking, high blood pressure, stress, pollution, and crowded cities. Yet the Japanese live longer than any other people on earth, and they enjoy relative immunity from heart disease.

If Japanese and Americans share the same bad habits and environmental stresses, why do the Japanese live longer? Scientists believe the answer lies in Japanese tradition, which fosters close personal ties to friends, family and community.

Studies here in the West lend credence to that theory. Increasingly, new research offers intriguing evidence that those of us who have richer relationships enjoy better health.

"Statistically, this is one of the strongest areas under study," says S. Leonard Syme, Ph.D., professor of epidemiology at the University of California at Berkeley and one of the world's leading experts on relationships. "What isn't clear is how it works. How does a relationship get into the body and influence biological processes? All we know at this point is, something very important is happening."

Dr. Syme, working with Lisa Berkman, Ph.D., wrote what many consider to be the definitive study on social ties and the risk of death. What Dr. Berkman and Dr. Syme discovered was compelling. They found that the socially isolated—the unmarried, divorced, or widowed, people with few close friends and few church or social contacts—were almost three times more likely to die of a wide variety of diseases than were people who enjoyed happy, fulfilling social lives. Without a safety net of close personal relationships, they discovered, we fall more vulnerable to disease.

Considering how lonely life would be without our friends and loved ones, the fact that they might also save our lives is an incredible bonus.

The Best Medicine

The Beatles, it seems, weren't far wrong when they sang, "Love is all you need." The best medicine we could possibly "take" doesn't always come in a bottle. Sometimes it flows through our relationships with the most important people in our lives. Finding ways to open up to these special people could be the single most important thing you ever do.

But it takes work. When it comes to building a deeper, more loving relationship, we need to learn and use some important skills.

Be Selective ● This is not to say some people are worthwhile human beings while others are not. But if you want lasting relationships, devote the most energy to the ones that matter the most to you.

"I'm a man with a cardiac condition, so I'm very impatient," says Gerald M. Phillips, Ph.D., professor of speech communications at Pennsylvania State University and coauthor, with H. Lloyd Goodall, Jr., of *Loving and Living.* "Time is very important to me. I won't waste time on people who annoy or bother me. You only have so much time on earth, so you might as well spend it on quality relationships."

Cultivate Candor ● When we were very young, openness was not a problem. We thought nothing of pointing to the man with the obvious toupee or telling the babysitter her braces looked funny.

As we grew older, though, our youthful candor went the way of the condor. But if we want to draw our friends closer, we'll have to save that endangered species, truth.

"The key to all relationships is honest communication," says Richard Grossman, director of the Health in Medicine Project at Montefiore Medical Center in the Bronx and author of *The Natural Family Doctor.* "So open up communication. Tell people what you really feel. It doesn't have to be a verbal message. It can be written. Send a letter. Call three friends you haven't heard from for a while. Take responsibility for communication. Openness is natural. We have the capability."

Know How to Use Small Talk ● If you're at a cocktail party and you're approached by a loud, opinionated political "expert," small talk is a handy way to dismiss him without hurting his feelings—if he has any.

As a preliminary to deeper, more meaningful conversation, though, small talk has a larger purpose. It's a reassuring ritual that lets you know that your friend cares about you, and vice versa. After "How's the job?" and "How are the kids?" you're free to discuss what's really going on in your life.

Put the Relationship First ● If husband and wife have conflicting needs—he wants a job in New York City, she wants to stay on the farm in Oneonta—both of you should consider what's best for both of you, not one of you.

This is one of the "trade secrets" of happily married couples, according to psychologist Florence W. Kaslow, Ph.D., president-elect of the American Psychological Association's Division of Family Psychology and director of the Florida Couples and Family Institute.

"There's a fine balance between, 'What's good for me' and 'What's good for the relationship,' " says Dr. Kaslow. Happily married couples manage to achieve that balance. "It's not only happy," adds Dr. Kaslow, "it's healthy. It's problem solving with a mutual concern."

Work Together ● You've probably noticed that some of your best friendships evolved out of a shared task, like building a treehouse at the local elementary school or planning a block party. "When I was a child, I lived in an area of the country that was prone to flooding," says Dr. Syme. "And I remember once, when I was about 11, working day and night for three days, filling sandbags for flood control, along with my friends and my neighbors. It was a highlight of my life. The best times I've ever had in my life were times I've worked with other people. It didn't seem to matter whether it was a good occasion or a miserable one."

Overlook the Warts ● "If the relationship isn't working, people think there must be something wrong with the person they're related to," says Dr. Phillips. "There must be a flaw."

But if the relationship is faltering, it could be because you have unrealistic expectations. You expect your friend, lover, or mate to be perfect. If you really want the relationship to grow, you should cut out the pedestal routine.

Share Everything — Even the Sad Stuff ● There's no rule that says we share only the good feelings and thoughts with our pals and mates. That's just half a loaf, and in this case half a loaf is no better than crumbs. When unhappy events bring you down, it can make you feel better just to share those feelings with someone who loves you. You aren't burdening anyone. In any case, your husband, wife, son, daughter, or best friend all know that when the world gets the better of them, you'll be there to hear their sad stories, too.

"Finding someone to share your weaknesses with is very important," says Dr. Phillips. "If you don't, you drown in them."

And that, he adds, is one of the most important things you need to know to take your sleepy relationships and turn them into something almost miraculously life-giving.

"I've had physicians tell me six times in my life, starting at age 11, that I had only a year to live," says Dr. Phillips. "I'm still here, I've proved all the doctors wrong, and I think that's because I have wonderful friends, all over the country, who help me along when I'm having a hard time. And they know that the love goes both ways. When they need similar treatment, they know they can cash their chips with me."

Turn Your "Twilight" into a New Dawn

There once was a time when the traditional props of old age were the rocking chair, the afghan, and a grandfather clock ticking away in the lonely, quiet distance. But that attitude is currently receiving a sound thrashing from Connie Goldman's radio series "Late Bloomer." Her guests, people over 65, can't remember the last time they saw a rocking chair, much less had the time to sit in one.

Consider Jacob Landers. Forced by a series of heart attacks to retire from his position as a school principal, he graduated from law school at 67 and is now a practicing attorney in New York. Then there's Thelma Tulane. Following the death of her husband, Thelma moved to a senior housing complex and at the age of 80 got involved with dancing. Now 88, she's touring schools, museums and community centers with a group called "Dancers of the Third Age."

"I've always been interested in aging," says Goldman. "After all, it's inevitable. The problem in this country is the stereotyped image that all old people are alike, that old age is like dropping off the face of the earth. What I've found during the production of 'Late Bloomer' is exactly the opposite."

"Late Bloomer" had its beginnings in Goldman's former job as an arts reporter for the National Public Radio Network. "While I was arts reporter, I became preoccupied with the positive attitudes of older creative people. Then, when I quit there, I founded a nonprofit business devoted to the production of educational, inspirational programs. My first series was called 'I'm Too Busy to Talk Now: Conversations with American Artists over 70.' "

During interviews with these people, the same message kept coming across. Sure, these artists were slowing down a little. Maybe an occasional midafternoon catnap was in order. But this was a reason to rearrange schedules, not quit. On the plus side, Goldman found these older artists to be very focused. "They know what they want to do, they bring years of experience to it, and they aren't sidetracked."

Happy with the positive tone and results of that series, Goldman decided to focus her energies entirely on aging. "I wanted to take the same concept as the previous series, only this time focus on what I call extraordinary, ordinary, older Americans."

The result was the "Late Bloomer" series, 65 separate five-minute interviews. The interviews focused on everyone, from millionaire to social security recipient, people of all races from all places. What these people have in common is that they've passed 65, made a change, and are having a great time.

The Turning Point

"I interview a lot of people who have faced the rocking chair," says Goldman. "They retired and then woke up on Monday realizing they had never really given much thought to what they would do next. The turning point for these people came when they assessed their abilities and discovered their true interests. And many times these interests had nothing to do with what they had been doing their whole lives."

A good "Late Bloomer" story illustrating this "changing horses in midstream" phenomenon concerns a post office employee and his wife who worked in a dress shop. Upon retiring from their jobs, this couple decided to move to Florida. They had no definite plans, but the climate was mild and friendly. One day while playing golf, the husband suffered a heart attack. His wife kept him going with mouth-to-mouth resuscitation until the ambulance arrived, and with additional attention at the local hospital, he pulled through.

The couple was so impressed with how nice the hospital staff had been that they decided to become volunteers at the gift shop and opened up a little sandwich bar there. Now they spend their early mornings gathering fresh vegetables, and from behind the counter they dispense healthy food, love, and comfort to the many anxious people who have friends and relatives in the hospital. What they make during their 60-hour work week goes to a scholarship fund.

If asked what attribute all these late bloomers share, Goldman would have to say a positive attitude. "I know it sounds a little trite and worn, but nevertheless it's true. No one ever said, 'Old age is so great we should all race and see who gets there first.' Each of these stories has a down side, whether it's an obvious one such as blindness or just a general lack of energy. But with these people it's not a matter of what their circumstances are, rather it's their attitude toward those circumstances. They're saying, 'I will not be beaten. I'm going to deal with the problems and win.' " Commitment also runs high among late bloomers.

A Writer's Late Start

One of Goldman's most amazing stories is about a woman who discovered her hidden talent at the age of 73. "Her husband had just passed away and there she was all alone in a big house," recalls Goldman. "She had always liked to read and now thought she'd give writing a try. So she found a writing class and began attending, although it meant a 30-mile night drive to the university. While the drive itself was an obstacle, even more difficult was the sometimes harsh criticism that went on in class." The woman is Harriet Doerr, who after a daily routine of writing and rewriting her material, went on to win the American Book Award in 1984 for *Stones for Ibarra.*

Currently, Connie Goldman Productions is working on another 260 "Late Bloomer" stories and will offer a cassette and book package entitled *Successful Aging: The Secret of How to Become a Late Bloomer.* The tape offers some of the success stories from Goldman's collection, while the book may give you some ideas and ways to get yourself started. Meanwhile, to hear the radio show and pick up five-minute packages of sheer inspiration, contact your local National Public Radio Station and ask them for a schedule.

Cultivate Your Courage Quotient

Who's risking more, the experienced parachutist who nonchalantly throws himself from an airplane or the little girl who swims across the deep end of the pool for the first time? The young man who joins a drug-smuggling ring or the one who becomes a Catholic priest? The woman who decides, finally, to get married, or the one with three children who gets divorced?

We all have our own ideas of what it means to take risks. If we're confirmed risk-takers, we may pride ourselves on our physical daring, inclination to take business gambles, or willingness to change hairstyle. If we avoid even the chance of risk, we may feel lucky simply to get out of bed each morning.

Most of us, though, are somewhere in between. We take some risks, but not as many as we'd really like. Fear makes us play it safe. We fear failure, embarrassment, bankruptcy, injury, or death. We feel a vague urge to shake things up, but often we're not sure exactly what it is we want or why we want to do it.

"Not the least of our problems is figuring out what 'risk'

means—to us, personally," says Ralph Keyes, author of *Chancing It: Why We Take Risks*. "Only when we understand the personal meaning can we know which risks we'd actually like to take."

Keyes, who conducts seminars on productive risk-taking for business and professional groups, defines a risk as something that causes fear and has the possibility of failure. The problem here, though, is that fear and failure are so subjective, and vary so much with time and circumstances, that only the risk-taker can determine what's genuinely risky. By this definition, someone who crosses the street despite being afraid of getting hit by a car is taking a bigger risk than someone else who leaps from an airplane with a parachute, sure of floating safely to the ground.

A simple test can assign weight to any apparent risk, Keyes says. "Simply add the word 'what' to a possible risk. Ask yourself what you are risking. Anything real? Anything valued? Something you would mind losing? Something you are aware might be lost? If you don't fear losing your life, is it a risk to play Russian roulette? If commitment to a relationship is a low priority, is getting divorced risky? If your financial base is secure, is it a risk to play the commodities market?"

And finally, he says, "Ask yourself, 'Do I care?' " Taking risks willy-nilly is not what we need, Keyes says. "We need a balanced diet of genuine risk, and we're the only ones who can assess what that means." The risks most people say they take aren't dramatic tales of mountain climbing or hang gliding. They are more likely to be things like confessing tender feelings to a loved one, speaking out on an unpopular viewpoint, or buying a home.

Why Take Risks?

Those who think risk-taking is vital to our well-being say it develops character and courage, extends our creativity, gives us confidence, and helps us establish a sense of limitations and possibilities. Risk-taking keeps us interesting and lively because we're occasionally willing to lay it on the line, to figuratively "expose" ourselves.

Some people apparently are natural risk-takers. The thrill of taking a chance gives them a biochemical "high"—a surge of neurochemicals that creates a state of extreme alertness followed by a pleasant calmness. Some people—criminals or compulsive gamblers, for instance—become almost addicted to the biochemical changes that come with risk-taking, says Marvin Zuckerman, Ph.D., a University of Delaware professor of psychology with a special interest in risk-taking.

"Sensation-seekers enjoy the heightened feelings they get when they confront fear," Dr. Zuckerman says. "People who go out of their way to avoid thrills may feel uncomfortable and overwhelmed by these sensations."

Fear Becomes Enthusiasm

It might seem that fear is keeping many of us from taking risks. In fact, the mountain climbers, tightrope walkers, and parachutists of the world say they're as scared as the rest of us. But they choose to act in the face of fear.

"In nearly every high-risk sport, the mastery of fear comes up repeatedly as the principal reward for engaging in it," Keyes says. One study found that the more frightened skydivers were while going up in the plane, the more enthusiastic they felt upon landing safely. In fact, the converting of fear into enthusiasm is so typical of the thrill-seeker that it may be a fundamental motive for courting danger, Keyes says. "Initially, you seek physical risk for the satisfaction of mastering your fear. In the process, you discover how exciting, even ecstatic, confronting fear can be."

First Steps to Risk-Taking

People who are unhappy because they seem to be naturally timid or who feel they're stuck in a rut can learn to take risks, one at a time, researchers say.

"Creating balanced diets of risk for ourselves and our families needn't mean that every item be a dangerous main course," Keyes says. "To the contrary, such menus ought to include appetizers and dessert as well.

"Putting more risk in your life might mean merely giving up a wristwatch to create the challenge of finding out what time it is. Or it could mean allowing yourself to follow a recipe only once. Or taking back roads instead of main routes, and not using a map. Or doing a jigsaw puzzle without looking at the picture."

And it also means looking at the larger risks you're taking now, and those you're doing a good job of eluding.

"The risks we don't take can be at least as interesting as those we do take," Keyes says. "In many ways, the risks we duck say something far more profound about who we are and how we feel than those we take. They speak to us of our deepest fears."

Keyes has even come to wonder if the risks we do take—authentic though they may be—are standing in for more profound risks we're avoiding.

"I think that when we do take a chance, no matter where it ranks on other people's scale of fear and risk, on our own, it's seldom at the top."

The weekend mountain climber, for instance, is taking a very real physical risk, but if he stopped to think about it, he might realize that he's using his alpine antics to avoid facing the reality of a deadly boring weekday job. He might decide a better future risk would be to look for ways to get into more interesting work. Keyes also cites the case of the woman novelist who signed up for an outdoors adventure trip rather than try her hand at writing a play. "She knew exactly what she was doing and what she wasn't doing," Keyes says.

The Risks Older People Take

Not surprisingly, people under age 30 score far higher on risk-taking behavior tests than do those over 30. Younger people tend to take many more physical risks; older people, with families and responsibilities, tend to take fewer physical risks. But they may take more mental risks.

"As risks become less frequent, people try to break out," says Frank Farley, Ph.D., a University of Wisconsin educational psychology professor. "A number of middle-aged people try to get involved in sports and physical activities they had put aside as they progressed in home life and career. But I think a good deal of this is more mental. If they are in a relationship that has really gone stagnant, they may get out of it. They might have affairs as a form of risk-taking."

In the interviews he did for his book, Keyes discovered that older people found it easier to take certain risks, like being open with other people, particularly people they cared about. He also discovered that those who stayed creative into old age seemed to become even more creative. They were willing to take more risks.

"The later years mean they are freer than they have ever been to adopt unorthodox concepts, and unorthodoxy is one of the recognized parents of creativity," Keyes says.

Those of us pondering a possible risk should note a final message from the many risk-takers Keyes interviewed.

"The greatest regrets I heard were not from those who had taken a risk and lost," he says. "Invariably, they felt proud for having dared, and even educated in defeat. The real regret, bordering on mourning, came from those who hadn't taken chances they'd wanted to take and now felt it was too late.

"For reasons ranging from the biochemical through the spiritual to the sexual, taking risks can enhance all our lives—even when the outcome is not as we'd hoped."

RATING THE RISKS

This is a test of risk-taking *tendencies* devised by seminar leader Ralph Keyes. There are no "right" or "wrong" answers, nor is any score "better" than another. Answer all questions, circling only one letter per question. If none of the answers given feels exactly right to you, pick the one that seems closest. Check your score below.

1. During the past ten years, how often have you changed residence? (*a*) ten times or more; (*b*) five to nine times; (*c*) two to four times; (*d*) zero to one time.

2. Which adjective best describes your behavior before age 12? (*a*) hyperactive; (*b*) mischievous; (*c*) basically well behaved; (*d*) very well behaved.

3. How often do you "put things off until the last minute"? (*a*) regularly; (*b*) often; (*c*) seldom; (*d*) almost never.

4. How often do you tape shut already sealed envelopes before mailing them? (*a*) almost never; (*b*) seldom; (*c*) often; (*d*) regularly.

(continued)

RATING THE RISKS — *Continued*

5. When eating Chinese food, how often do you use chopsticks? (*a*) regularly; (*b*) often; (*c*) seldom; (*d*) never.

6. In highway driving, how often do you drive faster than 65 mph? (*a*) regularly; (*b*) often; (*c*) seldom; (*d*) almost never.

7. If you were living on the East Coast a century ago, do you think you would have joined a wagon train headed West? (*a*) definitely; (*b*) probably; (*c*) probably not; (*d*) definitely not.

8. Suppose you had equal competence at any one of the following activities. Which would appeal to you most? (*a*) skydiving; (*b*) mountain climbing; (*c*) producing a play; (*d*) building a house.

For the following questions, assume that you are equally capable at all of the activities listed. *For each set,* pick the one that you would most enjoy. (If neither activity appeals to you, pick the one that's least unappealing.)

9. (*a*) driving a dune buggy; (*b*) hiking in the desert.

10. (*a*) skiing down a steep slope; (*b*) ski-touring through woods.

11. (*a*) scuba diving; (*b*) snorkeling.

For the following questions, choose the word that best describes your reaction to the activities listed.

12. Building a cabin: (*a*) tedious; (*b*) satisfying.

13. Climbing rocks: (*a*) exhilarating; (*b*) scary.

14. Attending a rock concert: (*a*) arousing; (*b*) jarring.

15. Teaching school: (*a*) boring; (*b*) challenging.

16. In a long-term relationship with someone you care about but with whom you're having problems, do you think it's best to (*a*) confront all of your problems at once, even though this might end the relationship; (*b*) confront some of your problems now, others later; (*c*) wait for a better time to confront any of your problems; (*d*) do nothing and hope that things will get better.

17. In general do you prefer the company of (*a*) people you've recently met; (*b*) professional colleagues, coworkers, or fellow members of a club or church; (*c*) old friends; (*d*) relatives.

18. Which opportunity sounds more appealing to you? (*a*) starting your own business; (*b*) purchasing a successful business.

RATING THE RISKS — *Continued*

19. Which statement describes you better? (*a*) I get bored easily; (*b*) When necessary, I can tolerate routine.

20. What kinds of risks would you say are hardest for you to take? (*a*) commitment risks (ones involving long-term involvement with a person, faith, activity, or career); (*b*) emotional risks (in relationships, or showing my feelings); (*c*) financial risks (of losing money); (*d*) physical risks (of life and limb).

Sprinter or Marathoner?

To determine your score, give yourself 1 point for each (*a*), 2 for each (*b*), 3 for each (*c*), and 4 for each (*d*) that you circled and total your points for all questions. A score of 30 or below indicates that you are more of a "Sprinter" when it comes to risk-taking. This suggests a high need for excitement and low tolerance for boredom. The hardest risks for Sprinters to take involve feelings and long-term commitments. A score above 30 puts you in the "Marathoner" category. While physical risks and those involving financial security may be harder for Marathoners, they have an easier time taking long-range risks such as raising a family or committing themselves to a career.

Whether it's preferable to be a Sprinter or Marathoner is a matter of taste and circumstances. Society would fall apart without Marathoners to keep things running. But some of history's greatest artists, explorers, and crisis-managing leaders have been Sprinters. Sprinters must pay more than the usual attention to choosing a vocation. For those with a high need for excitement, routine work can literally be unhealthy. Instead, they should consider working in a hospital emergency room, trading commodities, or starting a business. Managing existing enterprises is more suited to the temperament of a Marathoner. Their tolerance for routine and an ability to take the long view enables them to administer the enterprises that Sprinters start. Risking such long-term commitments is easier for Marathoners than Sprinters. But Marathoners are susceptible to understimulated lives. Marathoners have something to learn from Sprinters about taking short-term risks to keep their lives adventurous and nervous systems aroused. Without such short-term risk-taking

(continued)

RATING THE RISKS—*Continued*

they can have problems with lethargy and depression.

Problem areas for Sprinters include smoking, drug abuse, reckless driving, and petty crime. Their attention spans can also be perilously short. Developing a tolerance for the slow periods in any ongoing activity is important for them. Reading classic Russian novels may help, or learning to meditate.

Marathoners are better at risking such commitments but less good at making sure their lives include excitement and challenge. For Marathoners who enjoy outdoor activities, the wide range of physical adventures available to us today (such as kayaking or mountain climbing) can promote both physical and emotional health.

But there are many other ways to seek adventure. If the polls that have found that speechmaking is our most feared activity are accurate, giving a speech could be considered one of our most adventurous activities.

The ideal, of course, is to balance Marathons and Sprints in our lives: to combine family, career, and long-term friendships with regular opportunities for adventure, challenge, and daring.

The Healing Force of Laughter

"This is our specialty," says Ruth Hamilton, a grown woman, just before she pokes out her tongue and waves it enthusiastically to and fro. Next, she crouches down a bit, induces someone else to do the same, and they jiggle all four knees together. "We call it 'Humorous Yoga.'"

"We" is Carolina Ha Ha—short for Carolina Health and Humor Association—an organization cofounded and directed by Hamilton. The organization, unleashed on Durham and Chapel Hill, North Carolina, is serious about stirring up laughter. Carolina Ha Ha's proudest achievement of late is the

"Laughmobile," a cart disguised as a circus wagon, which brings funny cassette tapes, cartoon books, juggling parapher- nalia, bubbles, toys of every description—and spirited volun- teers like Hamilton herself—to patients in the cancer ward at the Duke University Medical Center.

Meanwhile, in Houston, Texas, humor and hope are dis- pensed together in an area of St. Joseph's Hospital dubbed "The Living Room." The room features not only a piano, a TV, and games and toys, but also "live acts"—stand-up comedians, magicians, and musicians. "It's designed to help patients coun- teract the negative emotions that go with their illnesses," says John S. Stehlin, M.D., surgical oncologist and scientific director of the Stehlin Foundation for Cancer Research at the hospital.

And in Albany, New York, the AIDS Council of North- eastern New York has just received a grant to explore ways that humor can help AIDS patients and the people who care for them. "I can just see people looking at the title of the book [we're writing], and saying, '*Humor and AIDS?!*'" says Alan Oliver, executive director of the organization. "But AIDS patients need the best possible coping techniques. They need stress reduction and to be more connected with people. And that's what humor does."

These days, a growing number of health professionals are talking about the importance of humor, laughter, and play for people who are ill, their families, and their caregivers.

"Laughter is a positive contagion that's spreading in the medical world, and other worlds," asserts Joel Goodman, Ed.D., director of the HUMOR Project at the Saratoga Insti- tute in Saratoga Springs, New York, and editor of *Laughing Matters* magazine. Dr. Goodman notes that about a dozen hospitals have set up humor and positive-emotion rooms, and many others have "humor carts" like the one at Duke. He points to the successful launching of organizations like Carolina Ha Ha and the American Humor Association. And, he adds, there are other telltale symptoms of this happy epidemic. "We've received grants to explore the uses of humor in thera- peutic situations. We've even been contacted by a medical school that is interested in integrating humor into their curriculum."

Laughter as Medicine

"Laughter is the best medicine" is an old expression, but it was former *Saturday Review* editor Norman Cousins in modern times who popularized the idea that there might be a direct link between laughter and health. In his book *Anatomy of an Illness,* Cousins describes how he recovered from a debilitating spinal disorder after a self-prescribed regimen that included a healthy dose of humor. He read humorous books and watched Marx Brothers films and "Candid Camera" episodes.

More recently, Cousins, now an adjunct professor at the University of California School of Medicine at Los Angeles, has said, "It is possible that laughter serves as a blocking agent. Like a bulletproof vest, it may help protect you against the ravages of negative emotion that assault you in disease. But I don't think we should ever take the position that laughter is a substitute for competent medical attention—I don't think there should be a conflict."

Dr. Stehlin concurs. "We are convinced that positive emotions have a lot of influence on the physiology of the human body. It's a difficult area to prove, but we're trying to see if we can document [whether] the positive reorientation will influence cells that are associated with the immune system. Because we do know that depression lowers the [effectiveness of the] immune mechanism. We are trying to work with the opposite of depression to see if it helps the immune mechanism."

So far, scientists have been unable to confirm any major physiological effects of laughter. But Alison Crane, a registered nurse and founder of the American Association for Therapeutic Humor, claims that there are numerous short-term benefits. Crane says that a good belly laugh may do nice things for breathing, blood pressure, muscle tension, digestion, and mood, though the impact may be mild and fleeting.

Perhaps even more important than the physical effects on health are the psychological benefits of humor and laughter, particularly for people who are ill or hospitalized.

Laughter Heals the Mind

"The hospital experience is by definition profoundly stressful," says Crane. "Humor can provide a distraction from the problems at hand, distance from things that can overwhelm us."

Sensitive use of humor can help, even in the most harrowing situations. Crane tells of one patient she was caring for, a 31-year-old man with a serious heart problem. Suddenly one morning, he began experiencing severe chest pain, and his condition rapidly worsened. The cardiologist decided that the man needed emergency surgery but felt he would get through it better if the man's wife and child—who lived an hour away—saw him before he went into the operating room.

"As the doctor was telling him what to expect, the patient's panic was rising to the point that he was almost incapable of talking," recalls Crane. "The family didn't arrive before he went down to surgery, so we had to keep his panic under control, and our own panic, too. My coping mechanism is showing humor. I had a gut feeling it would work, because we had a good rapport.

"So I tried to joke around—not as in gales of laughter, but just a little lightness to break the tension. For example, when hanging his IVs I put a baseball cap on his IV pole and said, 'This will be your friend for a while.' " The story has a happy ending. "The man came through with flying colors. A few months later, his wife wrote me, 'We cannot tell you how much your attitude before surgery meant. If you had not kept his panic down, he would not have made it.' Now, that may not have literally been true, but it *felt* that way to them. That means it was very important to their sense of well-being. Patients who are in pain are not going to be able to respond really well to humor, but they may appreciate it nonetheless."

Lenore Reinhard, coordinator of the Golub Humor Program at Sunnyview Rehabilitation Hospital in Schenectady, New York, says she knows that the humorous tapes and books they offer patients can help. "I remember a patient, a gentleman in his forties who was feeling a lot of stress. Relaxation tapes were not helping him. I suggested that he check out some of our humor tapes—we have Woody Allen, Bill Cosby, 'Father' Guido Sarducci, George Burns, Rodney Dangerfield, Mel Brooks, and others. Several weeks later, after he left, I checked the sign-out book—he'd borrowed *nine* humor tapes.

They really helped him relax and get his mind off the very difficult situation he was in.

"I remember another time," she says, "when I was new to the humor program, and somewhat naive, and I wheeled the VCR over to a group of stroke patients and asked them if they liked to laugh. One woman said, 'I used to like to laugh a lot, but I haven't laughed in a long time.' It was really special to turn on a segment of 'Candid Camera' for her and watch her reconnect with her sense of humor.

"Too often with patients, their illness becomes the focus," says Reinhard. "They must move from depression to acceptance, to getting on with it, and hopefully laughter expedites that process."

"I'm not saying people will get better 50 percent faster if they use humor," says Crane. "It's just that we're finding that humor programs really improve the quality of living in the hospital. Given the complexity of the health-care system, that's a big achievement."

Hawkeye Was Right

Just as people with illnesses can be helped by humor, so can their families and the professionals who care for them. Dr. Goodman first experienced the power of humor during his father's major surgery, when the lighthearted but sensitive man who drove Dr. Goodman to the hospital alleviated his fear and panic.

Now Dr. Goodman keeps a humor "first-aid" kit handy at all times. "I keep books of *Herman* cartoons next to my bed. Usually, if I'm down in the dumps, literally within two minutes I'm laughing out loud."

It doesn't always do the trick, adds Dr. Goodman. "In those rare times when I'm feeling down, I know that's part of the human condition—I don't avoid or deny that with humor. But I will use humor when I can to pick myself up."

Medical professionals, especially, need to learn to add humor to their lives. Hawkeye Pierce, Trapper John, Klinger, and the rest of the "M*A*S*H" gang knew the importance of laughter. "Front-line health-care professionals in particular deal with profound emotional and physical stress on a daily basis," says Crane. "Laughing at something frightening gives us a luxurious moment of distance. That's what "M*A*S*H" humor was all about—to keep those impossible, overwhelming things at the door."

Some health professionals, however, must be taught to bring humor into their own lives, says Dr. Goodman. "A large medical facility was having a problem with a staff that was in burnout. They brought me in for their first annual 'Staff Laugh.' Afterward, they wrote me that within 24 hours they had created a humor kit. It was a large wicker basket full of humorous books and tapes, kept permanently at a ward desk. Staff *and* patients can check out items whenever they need them."

But some health-care professionals know instinctively that laughter can be their own best medicine. Dr. Goodman recalls being told by a staffer at the Mayo Clinic about a one-liner from the *Wizard of Oz* that helped them cope. "When the going got rough, one of the staff would inevitably say, 'Toto, I don't think we're in Kansas anymore.' It worked wonders; they would all laugh and keep on going."

Help a Friend to Healthy Laughter

If you know a family member, a friend, or just a fellow human being who is ill or bedridden and realize that a prescription of joy and humor might help, you may wonder how to go about filling the prescription. Here are some tips from the humor experts:

● Remember that humor is not always appropriate. "When in doubt, I always try to use TLC (tender loving care) first," says Crane. "Listening skills and concerned compassion rarely fail. After that, use humor as an adjunct communications skill."
● Whenever possible, invite humor from the other person, rather than impose it on them. "Observe the person," says Dr. Goodman. "See what makes them laugh or brings joy to their eyes, and then try to invite occasions for that to happen."
● Take along cartoon books when visiting people who are ill, says Crane. "In medicine, we have a concept of unit-dose medication, putting each pill in its own package. I call the cartoon books like *Herman* and *The Far Side,* 'unit-dose comedy.'

You can open the books to any page, enjoy one cartoon and put it down feeling cheered."

● Encourage an older person to reminisce about happy memories or funny stories.

● If you know the patient well, don't hesitate to try the unexpected. "I have a number of friends who have been hospitalized and have had clowns deliver balloon bouquets or silly telegrams," says Dr. Goodman.

● Donate funny books or tapes to your local hospital. If you're looking for a more ambitious volunteer project, think about organizing a humor cart. Ruth Hamilton, of Carolina Ha Ha, says their 'Laughmobile,' which roams the hallways of the oncology ward at Duke University Medical Center, cost approximately $700. Most of the materials were donated—"fundraising is half of it," she says.

Massage Your Mind with Music

Music. Whether it's a snatch of Beethoven's Fifth on an aspirin commercial or five bars of "Dixie" honked out by the horn of a Ford pickup with Texas plates, we hear music every day of our lives. And the best part is, it comes in as many "flavors" as the ice cream from Baskin/Robbins.

Jazz, classical, bluegrass, pop, Irish reels, gospel—the list could go all the way down this page and up the next. As a matter of fact, there's probably a wider selection of music in your record collection than there are prescriptions in your medicine cabinet.

But while we've all managed to gain a little comfort from Bach or a spiritual lift from a sentimental tune, only in recent years has music been created specifically to benefit the body and mind. "New age" is the phrase currently used to describe this music. Almost always instrumental in nature and subtle and peaceful in form, it uses everything from bamboo flutes to acoustic harps and high-tech synthesizers. At the forefront of this new movement in music is Steven Halpern, Ph.D., author and composer of antifrantic music.

"There are times when you just want to put on some music, kick back, and really listen to it. That's fine," says Dr. Halpern. "But many times we have music playing in the background while we do other things, such as reading, cooking, or working around the house. Or we may turn on music to relax. Unfortunately, most music was just not designed for these situations and can actually get in the way of our original intentions.

"The foundation of western music, especially classical, is one of tension and release," Dr. Halpern explains. "As a passage steadily builds in intensity, your anticipation level builds with it. You're waiting for the big payoff, the release. And when the climax finally comes, the tension starts building all over again. But this time, you automatically start the cycle at a higher tension level." In effect, the music throws you into a state of tense anticipation.

New-Age Relaxation

New-age music is different. It doesn't lead you along an anticipatory path. Rather, it meanders along, slowly and unobtrusively, freeing your mind to wander. That has an overall relaxing effect.

If this is your first listening experience with new-age music, you'll need to acclimate yourself. Get comfortable, dim the lights, and let the music float you along. Feel it with your body and mind.

Do this for about 15 minutes the first time. After that, listen to the music whenever you like, for relaxation or even as background.

One thing you will notice is a lack of beat. "Any external beat sets up a rhythm entrainment in the body that literally takes hold and manipulates the heartbeat," explains Dr. Halpern. "Once, to demonstrate how external rhythms can force unnatural rhythms on the body, I asked a group of nurses to lie down on the floor and monitor their pulses while I pounded out a beat on the lecture stand. As I changed the beat, their pulses sped up and slowed down right along with me."

Certain new-age recordings, such as Dr. Halpern's "Spectrum Suite," lack an imposed rhythm and allow the body to choose the rhythm it finds most natural.

Considering the effects of rhythm and the anticipation response, it's easy to see how music, when not carefully chosen, can actually prove to be an annoyance. "Personally, I find that waking up to the wrong music makes me feel like I got only two hours of sleep," admits Dr. Halpern.

If you use a clock radio to sound the alarm, it really becomes a matter of pot luck as to what song starts your day. Fortunately, cassette alarm clocks allow you to choose your wake-up sounds.

"Basically, it's the difference between jumping into a cold lake and easing into a warm bath," says Dr. Halpern. "They both wake you, but one does it with a lot less stress."

Soothing Recordings

Whether you're looking for relaxing sounds, unobtrusive background music, or a way of masking some of the trying noises of daily life, new-age music offers a lot. And with consumer interest running high, record stores now have these selections in stock. Here are some of Dr. Halpern's favorites to get you on the road to a healthy listening experience.

- Kitaro: "Silk Road" (Canyon Records)
- Steven Halpern: "Dawn" (Halpern Sounds)
- Paul Horn: "Inside" (Golden Flute)
- Iasos: "Interdimensional Music" (Interdimensional Music)
- Emerald Web: "Valley of the Birds" (Bobkat Productions)
- Deuter: "Haleakala" (Kuckuck Records)
- Georgia Kelly: "Seapeace" (Heru Records)
- Paul Winter: "Common Ground" (Living Music Records)
- William Aura: "Auramusic" (William Auramusic)
- Mark Allen and Friends: "Summer Suite" (Rising Sun)
- Dallas Smith: "Stellar Voyage" (Rising Sun)
- Schawkie Roth: "You Are the Ocean" (Heaven on Earth)

- Daniel Kobialka: "Timeless Motion" (Li-Sem)
- Michael Stearns: "Morning Jewel" (Continuum Montage)
- Paul Warner: "Waterfall Music" (Waterfall Music Records)
- Environments: "Ultimate Seashore" (Atlantic)
- Solitudes: "Spring Morning on the Prairies" (Solitudes)
- George Winston: "Autumn" (Windham Hill)

Peace on the Home Front

Every day, the world bombards us with stress. That's why your home should be a haven, a place to balance yourself out and recharge your batteries. But that won't happen if your home life also happens to be stressful.

These tips from Paul J. Rosch, M.D., president of the American Institute of Stress, and other experts on the control of stress can remedy that situation and help turn your home into a center of regeneration.

Get Away from It All . . . Together ● If your partner won't talk or listen, having conversations with each other *outside* the home can be useful, says Kenneth Greenspan, M.D., of the Center for Stress and Pain-Related Disorders at Columbia-Presbyterian Medical Center in New York.

If the home is a stressful place, when you come home you may be conditioned to just shut off as a way to defend against stress. "Go out for dinner with your spouse, go away for the weekend or to some neutral setting," he says. "Don't try to solve your problems in the first minute. It should be more like, 'Let's go and enjoy ourselves and at the same time talk and be together.' Let things unwind a little bit. Do it on a day when you want to make as much peace as you can.

"Then when you talk, talk about what's right in the relationship first, then discuss what would be helpful to change. People get defensive and then they become unwilling to talk. And trying to make the other person feel guilty doesn't work."

Lean on a Friendly Shoulder ● "The feeling of being loved and cared for by friends and family goes a long way in protecting you from the negative effects of stress," says Nelson Hendler, M.D., a psychiatrist for the Department of Neurosurgery at Johns Hopkins Hospital and director of the Mensana Clinic in Baltimore. Surround yourself with people who will be there when the going gets tough. And give them the feeling that you will do the same for them.

Get a Handle on Finances ● Develop a plan to control spending and overspending. A big source of family stress is not how much money you have, but agreeing on how to spend it.

Take Control of Your Time ● Make daily "to do" lists. On each, rank four to six items in order of importance. Do them in that order, but don't fret if you don't finish everything. The only person who got all his work done by Friday was Robinson Crusoe. While you're making lists, make a "not to do" list of time wasters, such as meaningless TV shows and activities that you don't enjoy.

Put Things in Their Places ● Organizing your home helps you turn chaos into order. Designate a special place for all those items that you lose often. Place a special basket near the door for car keys, for instance.

Cool It, Then Say It ● "If you feel stressed because you can't control your partner's or your child's behavior, the first thing to do is to not let yourself get out of control, even though the things going on around you are very irritating and bothersome," says Dr. Greenspan. "Then once you have managed to control your own stress in this environment, see if you can communicate in a calm and controlled way. What happens very often is that one person's stress contaminates the other. So when you begin to have any kind of communication whatsoever, it breaks down very quickly."

Give Yourself Small Time-Outs ● Joel Elkes, M.D., director of the behavioral medicine program at the University of Louisville, says that you shouldn't let yourself become overwhelmed by tasks and obligations, but see them in perspective.

Set Appropriate Goals ● Accept what you can be and don't waste time worrying about what you can't be.

See Yourself in a Good Light ● List your strengths and skills.

Know That Wishing Won't Do It ● Stop yourself whenever you find yourself thinking, "If only I were rich . . . if only I had married someone else . . . if only I hadn't said what I did . . . " You may regret your mistake or your life situation, but living in the past or wishing for something you'll never have only stops you from reaching new goals.

Take the Word *Problem* Out of Your Vocabulary ● Replace it with the word *challenge.*

Stop the "Shoulds" ● Watch out for thoughts that start with "I should, I ought to, I have to, I feel obligated to, I owe it to him, I deserve." People often think they "must" do something, but what they really mean is that it would be "better" if they did something.

Watch Your Words ● Instead of saying "I can't *stand* your clutter all over the place," say "I don't like it." Whenever you escalate an "I don't like it" into an "I can't stand it," you are confusing your wants with your needs, which generates an incredible amount of stress. Most of the events or situations we think we can't stand are easily endured. Remind yourself that you can, and you'll spare yourself a good deal of stress.

Get the Facts ● Don't assume you know what another person is thinking and feeling. ("She's quiet because she's unhappy with our marriage . . . " "He's unhappy and it's all my fault.") Your reactions will likely be off base since they are based on assumptions, not facts.

Don't Overgeneralize ● Saying, "You never do what I want to do . . . you always do things the hard way . . . your mother never says a good word about me . . . men are all alike . . . women are all alike . . . all kids are maniacs . . . things never go right . . . nobody likes me," can create stress. Watch out for the words that overgeneralize, such as every, all, never, always, none, everybody, nobody.

Recognize Stressful Thoughts and Choose Not to Think Them ● You may think, for example, that a divorce or an unplanned pregnancy in your family may destroy your life, but you can learn to think of these "negative" things in a positive light. "Men are disturbed not by things, but by the view which they take of them," said Epictetus, the philosopher.

Don't Worry about Things That Are Not Worth Worrying About. ● In other words, "Don't sweat the small stuff, and remember, it's *all* small stuff," says Robert Eliot, M.D., a University of Nebraska cardiologist.

Laugh a Little ● Do not wait until all else fails to use humor. Laughter helps to ease anxiety, frustration, anger, and tension between people. Laughter may also help you tune in to optimism. There is evidence that laughter protects against the effects of negative stress by triggering the release of endorphins, the body's natural painkillers.

Give Family Ties Time to Bind ● "Don't work 20 hours a day and still expect to spend quality time with your family," says Dr. Hendler. "Cut back. And if your hours still don't permit enough time with your family, consider working flextime (going to work earlier and leaving earlier, for example) if that option is available to you."

Know That Trying for "the Good Life" May Not Be Conducive to Your Good Health ● Income isn't everything if your lifestyle is bringing you hassles instead of happiness. Take inventory and ask yourself if more family time wouldn't make you happier than a larger home that would mean more work, more commuting time to work and more bills.

If You Work, Try Not to Bring Your Problems Home at Night ● "I am convinced that the pattern of unloading daily stresses on friends and family bears an enormous risk," says Barbara Mackoff, Ph.D., author of *Leaving the Office Behind*. It is possible to use up their patience and concern. And the consequences may be anger, problems with your marriage, your children, or your love life—all from taking out your stress on your family. Leaving your cares at the office, on the other hand, may help you return to work refreshed and able to work better.

Destress before coming home, Dr. Mackoff suggests, by making "to do" lists, slowing down, asking to be alone for a while, requesting silence, exercising before getting home, exchanging stories about the funniest thing that happened that day, or identifying and connecting your feelings with the people and events in your day rather than pouncing on whomever you see first when you walk through your front door.

Eat, Play, and Work in Moderation ● Avoiding excesses is often overlooked as a way to prevent undue stress.

Examine Your Surroundings ● Is there too much noise, unpleasant odor, uncomfortable furniture, bad lighting, poor ventilation? Consider your options and don't overlook simple ways to take control over what you can control. Clutter, for example, can make you feel overwhelmed. A simple cleaning and clearing out can make you feel better.

Make Your House a Relaxing Place ● Does your bedroom feel welcoming at night? Maybe some fluffy new pillows would help. Can you bring spa comforts into your bathroom with a hot tub or a shower massage? Is your kitchen a place where friends and family feel comfortable sharing food and pitching in with the cooking? If possible, create at least one place in your home where you'll find it especially easy to relax.

Get Others to Share in the Housework ● If all adults in the household are working outside the home, hire all the help you can afford.

Don't Waste Time Trying to Be Perfect ● You can't expect to have the cleanest house, the whitest clothes, the most well-behaved children. Trying to be perfect can lead to burnout.

Treat Each Child as an Individual ● Children may bring not only joy to a home but also a significant amount of stress. For starters, to avoid contributing to their stress and ultimately yours, don't lump them together as "the kids."

Respect Children's Privacy ● Parents, for example, shouldn't go in and clean a child's room so he can't find anything. Negotiate with your child to clean his own room.

Assign Certain Tasks and Expectations ● Get it in writing. And let the children participate in the decision making. Being authoritarian and dogmatic doesn't work, says Dr. Hendler, father of four.

Have Clear Rules ● If fighting over toys is a problem, tell them, "If you keep it in your room, it's yours. If it's in the family room it's fair game."

Call a Truce in the Tub Wars ● If bathroom sharing is a problem, treat each other with consideration and set up a sequence of bathroom use in the morning. Establish a time limit when that's appropriate.

Plan a Special Outing ● If work is coming between you and your children, set aside time or make an appointment, if not for that day, then sometime in the near future when you will spend time together, says Dr. Greenspan. "Say that on Saturday afternoon, you will take one of your children to lunch or shopping. That goes a long way even though that child doesn't see much of you during the week. It's important for the child to know beforehand and not just have these events come up sporadically."

Work as a Team ● Hang up a family calendar. Hold meetings to juggle schedules. Block out time in advance for family activities.

Walk Away from Stress ● A massage or hot bath may do wonders to relax you. But don't overlook the benefits of a brisk walk or some other type of physical activity that you enjoy. Exercise, nature's tranquilizer, burns off excess adrenaline, the by-product of your body's response to stress.

Impatient? Breathe Deeply ● When waiting for an important phone call or when you're going to be late for your son's doctor's appointment because he's not home from soccer practice yet, take a few deep breaths. Expand the abdomen first, then the chest. When you exhale, collapse the chest first, then the abdomen. Learn to accept that it's no big deal to wait. Realize that trying to be in control is not helpful here, says Dr. Greenspan.

Make Relaxation Automatic ● Find cues or signals in your daily routine to remind yourself to breathe deeply and relax: before making a phone call, when the phone rings or whenever you wash your hands or brush your teeth.

Take a Relaxation Break ● "The Relaxation Response effectively protects people from the harmful effects of stress," says Herbert Benson, M.D., author of *Beyond the Relaxation Response.* "Anxiety and hostility often will disappear and you will be more open for changes of any sort, including even dietary changes or viewing the world differently." The Relaxation Response is the opposite of the body's response to stress. It decreases heart rate, metabolism, blood pressure and rate of breathing.

To practice the Relaxation Response, close your eyes and relax your muscles. Focus on your breathing. Breathe slowly and naturally. Select a prayer, phrase or word such as the number "one." Then repeat it or see it in your mind's eye each time you exhale. When outside thoughts intrude, disregard them by saying "oh, well" and return to the word or phrase you've selected. Always adopt a passive relaxed style in dealing with interruptions. Do this for 10 to 20 minutes once or twice a day.

A number of other techniques elicit the Relaxation Response, says Dr. Benson, including other kinds of meditation, breathing exercises, progressive muscular relaxation, and using special tapes or prayer.

In a Pinch, Don't Forget to Smile ● Stress-management programs often don't transfer to the scene of the crime, says Charles F. Stroebel, M.D., Ph.D., medical director of Stress Medical Clinic of Hartford and author of *QR: The Quieting Reflex.* When you're in a hot spot (in the middle of a big argument, for example), try using the Quieting Reflex: Smile inwardly and outwardly with your eyes and mouth. Say to yourself "amused mind, calm body." Take an easy, deep breath. While exhaling let your jaw, tongue and shoulders go limp. Feel a wave of heaviness come over your limbs and muscles. Feel warmth flowing through your body from your head to toes. Especially imagine warmth flowing into your hands. Then resume your activities.

"This is faster than popping a pill and you can do it anyplace, anywhere, anytime," says Dr. Stroebel.

Ask the Experts ● If you need further help coping with the stress in your home life, you may benefit from counseling or a stress-management program targeted for your specific problem. If you can't identify the exact source of your stress, make a list of the problems at home and physical symptoms that accompany them.

Then you can decide what you can and can't do about it, says Dr. Paul Rosch. Or you can take a test to identify and measure your stress. One of the most useful, the Seven Minute Stress Test, can be found in *The Doctors' Guide to Instant Stress Relief.* A longer version, the Stress Vector Analysis, is available from Medicomp, Inc., 1805 Line Ave., Shreveport, LA 71101, and may be included in many stress-management programs.

Some tips printed here come from Stresscare Systems, a stress-management program that is reviewed by a distinguished panel of physicians and scientists. For more information write to Stresscare Systems, Inc., 1000 Northern Blvd., Great Neck, NY 11021.

The American Institute of Stress is a nonprofit organization dedicated to furthering scientific investigation and knowledge of stress and health. If you have a question about stress or the appropriateness of a particular stress-management program, the American Institute of Stress can give you the latest scientific information and evaluations. They also publish a monthly newsletter containing current abstracts on all stress-related subjects. For further information, write to the American Institute of Stress, 124 Park Ave., Yonkers, NY 10703.

From there you can decide what type of stress-reduction program will benefit you most—such as biofeedback, family or career counseling, assertiveness training or counseling to change specific behaviors or bad habits.

Media Madness: Don't Let the News Get You Down

Policeman caught selling cocaine! Drug use among police officers rising! Fire in a warehouse! Suicide in a subway station! Child falls from 17th-story window and lives! Corruption in City Hall! Beirut death toll rises! London's worst fire since 1982! Two airliners nearly collide over the Atlantic!

Weather. Sports. Finally, the good news: This year marks the 40th anniversary of the bikini bathing suit!

And that's the way it was, according to a recent 10:00 P.M. local TV news program. Okay, this particular program *was* aired in New York City, a market renowned for its lurid appetite. But almost anywhere in the country, if you open the newspaper, or especially if you switch on the TV or radio news, the lineup isn't likely to be much more encouraging. Inexorable as the tides, the media sends out waves of this stuff every day.

How do you react to the daily tidings of tragedy? The bad news can present psychological dilemmas. Psychologists say that people's reactions are as diverse as their personalities. Some people may be haunted for days by major catastrophes—

like the space shuttle Challenger accident—or "minor" ones, like the murder of a distant stranger. On the other hand, there are the people who let it all roll right off them.

Is there a healthy way to respond to the bad news? Have you ever wondered if it's possible to be a well-informed citizen without having ice water running through your veins, or alternatively, being afraid to leave the house? And is the problem with the world, the news media, or with ourselves?

When these and other questions were asked of journalists, psychologists, and media critics, there was plenty of disagreement about the answers. But all agreed that through deeper understanding of the news media—and of our own reactions—we can find a better way to deal with the news and the bad news.

What's News?

"People everywhere confuse what they read in newspapers with news," essayist A. J. Leibling once wrote. He was, of course, referring to the vast difference between everything that happens on the planet and the particular events that editors select for use in newspaper, magazine, or broadcast.

In choosing from billions of possibilities, there's no doubt that the media tend to go for the jugular. Why is bad news considered more newsworthy than good? "News is something that deviates from the norm, and that's very often unpleasant," says television news consultant Jim Thistle, associate professor and acting director of the Boston University School of Journalism.

The importance of exposing people to the worst was proved in recent years by the war in Vietnam, Thistle argues. "The horror of Vietnam was plunked into people's living rooms, and people said, 'We shouldn't be in this war.' Television is credited with turning people around on Vietnam."

Of course, much of the bad news that the media choose to emphasize—the "Dog Bites Baby" stories—doesn't even approach the significance of Vietnam. Competition for readers or audience means media choose to "titillate instead of illuminate" with trivial but gripping footage or headlines of warehouse fires and freak accidents.

Of course, the news media isn't entirely to blame. Psychologists point out that the media wouldn't dish it out—the endless replays of Christa McAuliffe's parents' reaction to the Challenger explosion, for example—if the public didn't want to consume. "I think there's a certain attraction to being emotionally aroused by the news," says psychologist Tom Cottle, Ph.D., popular cohost of a morning television talk show in New England. "I wish I could get a nickel for everybody renting a horror movie tonight. We love to be frightened."

The result of the public's taste for thrills, and the media's race for ratings, is summed up in a particularly cynical newsroom adage: "If it bleeds, it leads." Paradoxically, the bad news that fascinates many people may also undermine some people's psychological well-being. Sonya Friedman, Ph.D., psychologist, radio host and author of numerous best-sellers, including *Smart Cookies Don't Crumble* and *A Hero Is More Than a Sandwich*, says she witnessed plenty of news-induced depression among single women a couple of years ago, in the wake of a media brouhaha over a study contending that women over 30 have little chance of marrying.

"One of the leading factors in the deterioration of mental health is the feeling of a lack of control," says Dr. Friedman. "That's why cataclysmic events, like earthquakes, or AIDS, or some study telling women that looking for a man is a dead end, have such a big impact. We feel totally undermined."

The feeling of lack of control develops not only because the items that the media report are so terrible but also because they are presented in a fragmented way, says Neil Postman, Ph.D., professor of media ecology at New York University and author of *Amusing Ourselves to Death: Public Discourse in the Age of Show Business.*

Television news is particularly bad in this regard, he contends. "The problem with TV news is that the language that usually accompanies the pictures is minimal, and it does not linger long enough to provide context. It seems to be a mélange of isolated, meaningless events.

"I think the most pleasing part of the news of the day is the weather, because at least if the man says, 'There's a snowstorm brewing in Texas, it's moving east and will reach Boston on Thursday,' you have a sense of continuity. It gives you a feeling, not of potency, but of understanding what the forces of nature are all about."

But most of the bad news is explained so badly, says Dr. Postman, that "I think the overall psychological effect is to increase the sense of impotence; that in the end there's nothing we can do except go back to the kitchen and get another piece of apple pie."

The Eye of the Beholder

Then there's a slightly different school of thought that contends that the fault, dear public, is not so much in the media but in ourselves.

"Basically, the news media do a pretty good job. It's people's irrational and crazy ideas and perceptions that tend to create misery," says Barry Lubetkin, Ph.D., clinical psychologist and director of the Institute for Behavior Therapy in New York City, the nation's largest private behavior therapy clinic.

"I find from my practice that people's response to bad news, and news in general, is very highly correlated with the way they handle life issues," says Dr. Lubetkin.

He cites some of the unhealthy responses of his clients to bad news.

● Personalizing. "Whatever the bad news is, they hook it up to themselves, rather than recognizing it as a random coincidental event that has nothing to do with them. It confirms the pessimistic, depressed outlook that they have anyway."

● Phobias. "Sometimes you will see fear of crowds, fear of subways, fear of dark places develop." Dr. Lubetkin notes that after the Challenger explosion, "a number of phobics seemed to get worse, particularly airplane phobics. They thought, 'If with all that scientific expertise, the Challenger blew up, how can I trust an airplane that gets much less scrutiny?' "

● Numbness. "Then there's the group that numbs out," says Dr. Lubetkin. "They hear bad news, or read it, but they put on blinders and earplugs and remain indifferent."

● The wild response. "There's another group that somehow uses bad news to justify carrying on their lives in a wild way.

They say, 'What the hell, the world's going to pot anyway, let me just enjoy myself and act without conscience.' "

● Charmed. "Some people welcome the randomness of violence—not that they look forward to it, but they tend to believe they lead a charmed life. The randomness of bad news allows them to continue with the illusion that nothing can touch them, that they'll always be in the right place at the right time."

What's a better response? "Probably the most adaptive response is what I call reasonable vigilance," says Dr. Lubetkin. "That means these people think, 'The world is unpredictable, the world is basically unfair, it metes out bad and good luck independently of what I hope, pray, dream, or desire. I have to accept this as a basic reality of life. I will be reasonably vigilant, I won't pick up strangers hitchhiking, but I accept a certain amount of risk, which is part of being a human being.' "

For patients who do have inappropriate news-related phobias or anxieties, Dr. Lubetkin recommends a technique called relabeling. "Relabeling is challenging irrational beliefs," he explains. Patients who were nervous about flying in the wake of the Challenger tragedy, for example, were helped by focusing on all the planes that take off and land successfully each day.

Good News Is No News?

Isn't it simpler just to turn it off? Joyce Anisman-Saltman, a Connecticut psychotherapist and sometime comedienne who teaches executives and clients all over the country how to put more laughter in their lives, wholeheartedly endorses this approach. "Every time I'd read the newspaper, I'd go, 'Tsk, tsk,' 'Oh my God,' 'Honey, did you see that?' 'Isn't this terrible!' "

So she went cold turkey—she simply no longer reads or watches TV news. As evidence that this technique works, Saltman points out that vacationers usually don't read the newspapers. "When we're trying to recharge ourselves, we instinctively stop reading the newspaper to feel better. I accept that one of my shortcomings is that I'm not a well-informed person. I'm good at other things," she adds.

There are two problems with the cold-turkey solution.

First is our responsibility as citizens of a democracy to stay informed. And second is, as Dr. Lubetkin puts it, "You can't turn it off forever."

Fortunately, there are plenty of other things you can do to deal with the news in a better way.

Be a Choosy Consumer

The first step is to be a choosy news consumer and recognize that all news sources are not alike. Television is more explicit than newspapers and tends to aim for the emotions rather than the mind.

If you do watch TV news, you may want to opt for the 6:00 P.M. version rather than the later shows. News consultant Jim Thistle points out that news directors are looking for a fresh lead on the later show, and are more likely to opt for a dramatic-but-not-very-important crime or fire. The morning news tends to be the most "user-friendly," Thistle adds.

Most experts say that, in general, newspapers are a better choice than TV or radio, because they have space for more explaining. Some newspapers are more responsible than others, though. And selective reading of your favorite newspaper may also be necessary. As one eminent journalist put it, "A headline is not an act of journalism, it is an act of marketing." If the headline reads, "Ax Murderer Strikes Again"—and you know it will upset you—you don't have to "buy" the story by reading it.

Psychologists emphasize that there are many ways to consciously adopt a healthier attitude to the bad news. "Take whatever you read and diminish your reaction by one-half," says Dr. Friedman. "Then ask yourself whether you have any control over the situation, whether you can make a difference. If the answer is 'no,' you must recognize that that is one part of civilization you are not a factor or participant in, and which will roll along without your involvement.

"But if there is any way your involvement—a vote, a letter, a donation—can make a change for the better, you owe it to your mental health to do that, to take control," adds Dr. Friedman.

Challenge Your Mind
and Recharge Your Life

Constant intellectual stimulation is important to psychological and physical well-being. This was tellingly illustrated in a public television documentary that dealt with primate behavior in a zoo that provided the animals with very little stimulation. Basically, orangutans, chimps, and gorillas derive a great deal of their stimulation in captivity through jungle-gym-like climbing structures, which approximate their tree-covered natural homes. At Granby Zoo in Quebec, the only thing the primates had to play on were some very simple, time-worn poles providing little of the intellectual stimulation they required. Naturally, just like humans, the apes grew bored.

What was interesting was the disruption of their natural behavior patterns when they did not receive the stimulation they needed. Some paced restlessly about their compound. Others grew aggressive toward tourists as well as their own kind. One chimp even lost all sexual desire.

Think about that the next time you're bored!

When new and complex structures (a cross between a glorified treehouse and a ship mast's rope riggings) were built for them, the apes gradually reverted back to some of their natural behavioral patterns and exhibited signs of contentment.

Just as a chimpanzee needs climbing toys, and mice need dirt in which to burrow, we too have our DIR (daily intellectual requirements). But what *is* our DIR? The importance of this question is highlighted by the fact that the brain is our primary tool of survival.

The main point of regeneration is not merely to squeeze a few extra years out of life. Striving for excellence, the adventure of discovery and the realization of our latent potential are the true targets. Look for these and a longer, happier life becomes a bonus.

Are You in a Groove or in a Rut?

All that sounds easy enough, but it's just as easy to fall into stagnation. A typical image of boredom is two kids with their chins in their hands, watching a rainy day through the living-room window. In fact, boredom is much more insidious. It can sneak up on you even in the midst of a busy life. You might be doing your daily business, making conversation, going to restaurants, and feeding your pet flamingo . . . but suddenly it all just ain't tootin' your horn anymore.

Question: When does a groove become a rut? Answer: Imagine driving to the same place every day. The first few times, you get lost, drive slowly, and get a little edgy trying to find the place. After a while, you learn the route. You relax and enjoy some of the scenery along the way. Now you're in a groove. But as more time goes by, you do the drive by rote. The scenery goes by unnoticed and the trip no longer is a source of stimulation. Now you're in a rut.

The analogy can be transferred to just about any aspect of your life; home, office, relationships. To avoid a rut, one of two things must be done. First, you can change the activity or the circumstances. Rearrange your furniture or drive a new way to work every other week. Even simple things like these can have their effect.

Second, if the activity can't be altered, change your perspective. You can't change jobs or spouses every time you think you're in a rut. But try looking at and appreciating what you're doing from a different viewpoint. It's rather like watching the same movie with a different sound track. It'll *feel* like a new movie. One couple tried changing their sound track when dinnertime conversation was getting a bit lax. They pretended not to have known each other for the past ten years. As they asked each other questions that hadn't been asked since before their marriage, they found they were both getting new and unexpected answers. Playing strangers allowed both of them to see a new person hidden inside the other.

The Healing Power of Walking

Walk for Your Heart's Sake

If you're in need of some inspiration to "keep up the good walk," get ready to beat feet. A major study has just confirmed what other studies have suggested all along: *Every step you take is a step toward a stronger heart and a longer life.*

Some 12,000 men who were at risk for developing heart disease participated in the study. During seven years of follow-up, researchers at the University of Minnesota School of Public Health found that those men who were moderately active in their leisure time had 30 percent fewer deaths from heart attacks than more sedentary men (*Journal of the American Medical Association*).

In particular, the decreased chance of dying was associated with light- and moderate-intensity activities: that is, walking— and also bicycling, fishing, bowling, gardening, yard work, home repairs, dancing, and swimming, for example. And the duration of activity necessary to make a difference was only 30 to 69 minutes a day, the researchers report. "This is an encouraging finding . . . since most people should be able to schedule this amount of time for physical activity as part of their daily routine," they say.

This is not the first time scientists have seen this effect. In an ongoing study of Harvard alumni, researchers found that men who burn 2,000 or more calories a week in walking, stair climbing or sports have a 28 percent lower death rate than those who do little or no exercise (*New England Journal of Medicine*).

The Minnesota researchers think that the main reason for the lower death rate in more active men is the effect of improved physical fitness on the heart. Studies show that a regular walking program lowers blood pressure and resting heart rate. And it improves aerobic fitness, the ability of the body to use oxygen.

Walking decreases levels of artery-clogging blood fats while increasing the level of high-density lipoprotein (HDL), the beneficial kind of cholesterol. And walking helps make the heart muscle stronger.

Many studies suggest that walking can help prevent a second heart attack in people who've already experienced one.

Other Body Benefits

But the benefits of walking don't stop at a healthier heart. Among the other reasons to keep in step:

Weight Control ● Exercise may also lead to a longer life by helping people maintain their proper body weight, say the Minnesota researchers.

Exercise is an important component of any weight-loss program. And walking is particularly well suited to the task because it is so gentle. The last thing an overweight person needs is an exercise that pounds his joints.

Walking revs up your metabolism so you burn more calories. And it increases the burning of body fat, not muscle. That's important because muscle tissue burns more calories. The more muscle you lose, the harder it is to burn calories. Walking may also help curb your appetite.

Mood Elevation ● Walking can lift your spirits by stimulating the release of natural mood-elevating chemicals called endorphins, studies show. And some researchers have found it helpful in easing depression. In a study at the University of Southern California, researchers found walking to be more effective than a tranquilizer in relieving anxiety.

A brisk walk steps up blood flow to the brain, making for clearer and more creative thinking, some studies suggest.

Walking is a social activity—you can do it with a friend and enjoy the company. And there's no question that the feeling of accomplishment at having sustained a regular walking program is a real confidence builder.

Stronger Bones ● Bones need exercise, too. They respond to weight-bearing exercises, such as walking, by taking on more calcium. They can become thicker, stronger, and more resistant to osteoporosis. Some studies show that the progression of osteoporosis is slowed by regular exercise.

A Pain-Free Back ● Walking can help relieve back pain by strengthening and toning muscles that make the spine more stable. Unlike running, it puts no more stress on spinal disks than standing, and less stress on back muscles than sitting.

Increased Energy ● A brisk ten-minute walk can make you feel more energetic than the often-touted candy bar can, reports a researcher from California State University. Robert E. Thayer, Ph.D., found that the energy boost from walking not only kicked in sooner but also lasted longer. And the people in the study were less tense after the walk than after the sweet treat.

A Whole-Body Tone-Up ● Your legs, hips, buttocks, and lower abdomen all see action in walking. As you pump your arms, they get a workout, too. So do your shoulders and forearms, sides, back, and chest. The vigorous breathing expands your chest and lungs and gets your diaphragm working.

Walking has been shown to act as a good substitute for cigarette smoking, to help alleviate headaches in some people, and to discourage the onset as well as the progression of varicose veins.

How's that for inspiration?

The Exercise/Cancer Connection

Could being physically fit help prevent cancer? Nobody knows for sure, but recent studies suggest an intriguing association for some kinds of cancer.

Take breast cancer, for example. Researchers at Harvard University found that women who had been active in basketball, swimming, tennis, track, gymnastics, volleyball, or other sports in college later developed significantly less breast cancer than their inactive peers. Their sedentary classmates had twice the risk for breast cancer as well as 2½ times more cancer of the uterus, ovaries, cervix and vagina.

And take colon cancer. Three separate, large population studies published in the last four years have found that men with physically active jobs, such as carpenters, plumbers, gardeners, and mail carriers, have an advantage. They are much less likely to develop colon cancer than accountants, lawyers, bookkeepers, and other workers who merely shuffle papers and push pencils.

Of course, researchers say these studies don't prove that exercise helps prevent cancer. They *do* say, though, that the few studies done so far have all reached the same conclusion: that physically active people get less of certain types of cancer. That evidence has been enough to convince the American Cancer Society to recommend exercise as one possible way to reduce the risk of this killer disease.

What Research Can Show Us

In some ways, animal studies can demonstrate a clearer association between exercise and cancer than human population studies. "With animals, we can control most of the variables that could confound population studies," says Leonard Cohen, Ph.D., head of the section of nutrition and endocrinology at the American Health Foundation in Valhalla, New York.

Researchers know mice aren't going to smoke cigarettes or stay up all night drinking and playing cards—complicating variables that can skew the results in human studies.

In a study by Dr. Cohen, rats were given a chemical that induces breast cancer. Then, half the rats were put in cages that allowed them free access to an exercise wheel. These rats could run anytime they wished, and they did so frequently.

"It's important to stress here that the *only* difference between the two groups was the exercise wheel," Dr. Cohen says. "The rats with access to the wheel developed one-third fewer cases of cancer than the inactive rats. And the tumors appeared much later in the active animals."

What does this all mean? "There seems to be some good evidence that exercise reduces your chance of getting breast cancer, and possibly other cancers, by means which we don't yet understand," Dr. Cohen says. "More questions need to be answered before we can confirm the cancer/exercise link." In fact, studies of this sort are under way at this moment.

The Body-Fat Link

Researchers think one reason exercise may protect against cancer is that it whittles away body fat. They've noted that overweight women get more cancer of the uterine lining, and, in postmenopause, tend to do less well once they have breast cancer.

How does body fat relate to cancer? Fat seems to have a direct effect on a woman's hormones. "The fatter you are, the more you convert androgen [a male hormone] to estrogen [a female hormone]. Also, more of the estrogen is metabolized to a potent form. This may explain why excessive fatness is a risk factor for breast and reproductive cancers," says Rose Frisch, Ph.D., of Harvard, who conducted the study of former female college athletes. "Estrogen stimulates cells to divide in the breast and reproductive system, particularly the uterine lining. So excess or too-potent estrogen could be implicated for cancerous growth." Lean women also produce less of a hormone called prolactin, which stimulates cell growth in the breasts' milk ducts, a very common cancer site.

In colon cancer, researchers are less sure what role body fat plays, but they think it might involve the body's manufacture of prostaglandins. These potent biochemicals are made from fats. Some cause an inflammatory response, which might be linked with cancer development.

Constipation, too, has been linked with colon cancer, and there's evidence that inactive people are more likely to be constipated. Exercise stimulates the peristaltic action of the intestines that results in regular and more frequent bowel movements. This may shorten the time that cancer-promoting materials remain in contact with the intestinal lining.

Changes in eating habits may also be involved, says John Vena, Ph.D., of the State University of New York, Buffalo. Researchers have found that, for whatever reasons, athletes tend to eat more low-fat, fiber-rich complex carbohydrates, such as bread and pasta, than inactive people. Those foods could help protect against cancer, Dr. Vena says. Athletes are also much less likely to smoke cigarettes or to drink heavily, but population studies usually try to take this into account.

Exercise can easily cause a temporary negative energy balance. It can force the body to dip into its energy reserves, converting stored protein into usable glucose. Some researchers think that hormones used to initiate this process, glucocorticoids, provide the body with cancer protection. "In experiments with rodents, treatment with glucocorticoids retarded the development of a number of cancers, including mammary and skin cancer," says Michael Pariza, Ph.D., of the University of Wisconsin. "And we know that glucocorticoid levels can go up during exercise.

"But there are still many questions about what type of exercise is best and the extent to which exercise can really help people."

Researchers have also noted that, in a number of animal studies, food restriction leads to reduced rates of cancer, while free access to food leads to increases. They think glucocorticoids are involved. "It's thought that exercise may reinforce the favorable hormonal changes that occur during modest food restriction," adds Dr. Pariza.

Aerobics for Immunity?

Several studies have indicated that exercise stimulates the body's cancer-fighting immune system. In some of the studies, exercise increased numbers of potential cancer-fighting white blood cells called lymphocytes. In others, it boosted levels of lymphokines, chemical messengers that rally lymphocytes to action.

In studies in the United States and England, bicycling, running, and stair climbing increased the numbers of lymphocytes circulating in the blood. Lymphocytes known as natural killer cells are one of the body's first defenses against cancer. They can kill certain tumor- and virus-infected cells.

In an Italian study, blood levels of interferon, a virus-fighting substance, more than doubled in men who rode bicycles for an hour at a moderately intense pace.

And in a study from Tufts University School of Medicine, levels of interleukin-1, a biochemical that stimulates proliferation of lymphocytes, increased in men after an hour of moderate bicycle riding (*Journal of Applied Physiology*).

Just how does exercise work in these cases? No one really knows. It may cause an inflammatory reaction in the muscles, to which the body responds by sending in lymphocytes. Exercise also breaks down a small number of red blood cells, which means that lymphocytes could be sent into the bloodstream to clean up the pieces.

Endorphins, those "feel-good" biochemicals that runners say get them high, may also play a role. Endorphins might create changes in the endocrine system that may have a cancer-inhibitory effect, Dr. Cohen says.

The big question—whether exercise boosts immunity enough to ward off cancer—is not yet answered. There is still no real proof that it can prevent cancer or that it's useful in treating cancer.

Have Fun, Take It Easy

Before researchers can recommend how hard or how much you should exercise, more studies need to take place. In animal studies so far, moderate activity seems to work better than extremely intense exercise. Animals forced to exercise at a relatively high intensity on a constantly moving treadmill or in a tub of water actually have increased cancer rates.

"The animals in my study are walking fast. But they are not panting," Dr. Cohen says. "They are very relaxed and docile, having a good time. They stop when they want, and they go when they want."

One of the biggest pluses for exercise might actually be its ability to relieve stress, Dr. Cohen and other researchers agree. "I'd tell people to find a physical activity that leaves them relaxed and happy."

"There are already so many good reasons to exercise, preventing cancer could be just one more," adds Dr. Vena.

Let a Daily Walk Do Your Dieting

Hello, class, welcome to today's advanced seminar on walking and weight loss, in which we explore how walking helps you slim down and shape up and. . . .

Yes? You have a question? You say you've been walking ever since you were knee-high to a bathroom scale and haven't dropped an ounce? In fact, you've been *gaining* weight for years? And you want to know how something as easy and natural as walking could possibly have an impact on something as stubborn and immovable as flab?

Those are good questions. First of all, this class isn't on "walking," as in, "I think I'll walk over to the couch now." This is about *walking*—deliberate striding that's sustained (generally 30 minutes or more) and regular (three to six times a week) and paced (a clip that's comfortable but brisk).

Second, science assures us that this kind of walking can exert enormous power over mind, muscle, and fatty matter.

Especially the latter. In fact, research has suggested at least six ways that the simple pace beats pounds of pudge.

Walking Proud ● Feeling down and out can undo any weight-loss program. But walking is a blues buster. Through hormonal sleight of hand, it can elevate your mood. And through the feeling of accomplishment it gives you, it boosts your self-image and self-esteem.

Good Burn ● People sometimes forget that walking rivals running as a calorie burner. If you weigh 150 pounds and walk a brisk two miles, you'll expend 200 calories. Do that six days a week for a month (and keep your food intake constant) and you'll walk off 4,800 calories, or about a pound and a third of excess baggage. In a year you would drop almost 18 pounds!

Fast Burn ● Somehow brisk walking fiddles with your body's carburetor. For up to several hours after you stop walking, your body's normal burning of calories (the basic metabolic rate) gets stuck in fast idle, burning at a higher rate than before you walked. Faster burn means faster weight loss.

Deep Burn ● Walking not only melts fat, it also builds muscle (which looks better on you than lard any day). And, hour after hour, muscle tissue burns calories faster than fat does, an edge that can help you cut poundage over the long haul.

Diet Aid ● Walking, or any other exercise, doesn't rev up your appetite. There's evidence that it throttles it down, or at least puts it in neutral. That's why walking before meals is a great way to suppress the urge to gorge.

Less Stress ● A good long walk helps defuse stress and tension, which helps you beat the temptation to use ice-cream sundaes or chocolate fudge as tranquilizers.

Class dismissed. Let's go for a walk.

A DAY-BY-DAY, SAFE-AND-SANE WALKING PROGRAM

Your personal walking program begins in your head, not in your feet. So, first, think safety: If you haven't had a medical checkup in a while, get one. Think hardware: Invest in a superior pair of shoes—not just athletic shoes, but *walking* shoes. Skip the ones that have a so-so fit and buy those with the fit your feet will love. Then think commitment: Determine now to give your walking program at least a 30-day trial.

Day 1

Walk for 15 minutes straight—no more. Walk fast enough to hurry your breathing slightly but not so rapidly that you can't carry on a conversation. If this pace is too tiring, slow up. If it's too easy, shift gears. Lock in on your personal pace.

From here on out, you have to listen to your body carefully to modulate your walking schedule. On any given day, if walking the suggested number of minutes is a strain, fall back to the preceding day's schedule until it seems too easy. It's okay to go slower than this program indicates but never faster.

Days 2 through 6

At your personal pace, walk one minute longer on each consecutive day so that by the sixth day you're up to 20 minutes.

Day 7

On this day thou shalt rest without one little cubit of guilt.

Days 8 through 14

This week, walk six days and continue adding a minute each day onto your walking time until you're up to 26 minutes per walk. (But, if tacking on even an extra 60 seconds foments a revolt in your calves or shins or feet or anything else, drop back to your previous time for two or three days. And if trying to walk six days this week seems like it will be too demanding, go for five or four but no fewer than three.)

A DAY-BY-DAY, SAFE-AND-SANE WALKING PROGRAM — *Continued*

Days 15 through 21

Same as last week, except try to work up to a 32-minute walk. (If you lag behind this pace, no sweat. There's always next week. Besides, you're not racing anyone.) Also, nail down your schedule to three, four, five or six days of walking, whatever's comfortable to you. Create a routine that you can look forward to. From here on out, try to stick to this schedule, walking at the same time during the day.

Days 22 through 28

Stay on your regular schedule, 32-minute walks.

Day 29

Your walk has been cancelled. Today you celebrate your new-found fitness (and probably the absence of some blubber). Buy yourself a gift, take the day off, indulge yourself.

Day 30 and Beyond

You made it! Now you're a regular dyed-in-the-wool walker. If you keep it up, you'll have nothing to look forward to but better health, a livelier step and leaner looks.

Children's Health Updates

How to Get Monsters out of the Closet

Michael and Diane Veit spent about $2 to help their three-year-old overcome her fear of monsters. Every other night, a can of Lysol disinfectant moonlights as monster spray to keep invisible beasts out of their Cypress, Texas, home.

For Kim Adams, mother of a young son in Dobson, North Carolina, a real fears-away spray would have been only too welcome. "Jordan just recently calmed down about his fears of the dark, being alone, and monsters. Before that, he'd always come scampering to our bed at night, waking his sister and bringing her with him. He wouldn't even go to a different part of the house without me during the daytime. He handles things better now, but for a while we were really frustrated."

Whether they cause full-blown frustration or just pose an occasional problem, fears are as much a part of being a kid as lost teeth and security blankets. Still, when the vacuum cleaner is plugged in and your child heads (screaming) for cover, you can't help but wonder: Is my child behaving normally? Is there something I can do to help?

Experts agree: In the fight against fear, knowledge is power. Understanding the causes of childhood fears (*you* may be one!) will help you determine what coping approach will best work for your child. It may also help you head off some fears *before* they develop.

246

Setting the Stage for Fright

Some fears, we realize, are simply the Swiss army knives of emotions—practical, helpful in a pinch. We're glad our kids are afraid of cars when they're playing in the neighborhood, are afraid of heights when something dangerous is begging to be climbed. Sometimes we're fearful as a survival instinct—every baby is terrified at the thought of being abandoned. Other times, however, the appearance of a fear doesn't have such an obvious explanation.

Transferred Anxiety ● The reason for the pink balloons all over the house comes home from the hospital with you: the baby sister. Several weeks later, your normally tough-guy toddler is screaming about monsters chasing him in the middle of the night. More than a coincidence?

"Something upsetting that's happening in a child's environment can take on a more concrete form—such as a scary monster," says Alvin Poussaint, M.D., associate professor of psychiatry at Harvard Medical School and script consultant for television's "The Cosby Show." "Monsters become somewhat of a universal symbol to children who are feeling threatened, vulnerable, and unprotected, but who can't express why. Going to the day care center, parents fighting, and being 'replaced' by a new brother or sister are examples of concerns that can manifest themselves as monster fear, which is easier for a child to understand than the actual worry."

Generalizations ● For many children, one bad experience can increase the scariness quotient of the world tenfold. A painful sting from one bee often incriminates every creature that flies, crawls or slithers near the hurt child. One two-year-old boy now cries, "Car come and get me!" whenever he's upset. It's logical, since several months ago a pickup truck crashed through the wall of his bedroom in the middle of the night.

Temperament ● Parents curious as to why they have one fearful child and one unshakable trouper may have an explanation in research done by Edward Sarafino, Ph.D. "There may be a link between the temperaments that children are born with, and the development of fears," explains Dr. Sarafino, who is the author of *The Fears of Childhood* and professor and chair of the Psychology Department at Trenton State College in New Jersey.

"Children born with difficult temperaments—those who cry a lot, have irregular schedules, rarely sleep through the night, and don't adapt very well to new situations—are much more likely than children born with easy dispositions to develop a wider variety of fears, and more intense fears, later in life. It may also be that the way parents relate to these different personalities affects the fear capacity to come."

In addition, a shy, insecure child may be more susceptible to fears than a confident go-getter. "If a child feels incompetent and powerless, he'll naturally feel more anxious and fearful. When he's afraid of one thing, he thinks, 'Gee, if I can't handle being by myself, what makes me think I can handle darkness?' " Dr. Sarafino notes.

Although the amount of evidence suggesting it is small, one other theory points to a genetic contribution to how fearful a child will be.

Overprotectiveness ● More than once you may have rushed to pull your child off a chair she climbed, yelling that she'd fall and hurt herself. This behavior of yours can send a good message—safety—but if done often enough, it may hurt her more than a chance tumble to the floor. "If your child isn't allowed to try things out and take an occasional risk," says Dr. Sarafino, "she'll start to feel the world is a dangerous place, and all the things she's thinking of doing can get her injured. Consider how often we give warnings like these to children: Don't go near the water or you'll drown. Don't cross the street or you'll be run over. Don't lie or God will send you to hell. Don't look like you're afraid of the dog or he'll bite you. We can teach safety without always sounding this threatening."

The paranoia about kidnapping that's recently swept the country is another example of how being overprotective can spur a child's fears. Dr. Poussaint, who is also a senior associate at the Judge Baker Children's Center in Boston, tells of working in his clinic one day when a three-year-old girl walked in with her mother. "The little girl came right up to me, said hello, and shook my hand. Her mother whisked her away and scolded, 'Didn't I tell you never to talk to strangers?' And this was in a professional's office! The girl was only having a normal play interchange with me, but her mother made her feel just being friendly was a dangerous thing to do."

Several other things can also make children fearful. Sometimes parents try to squelch bad behavior with threats of "If you don't stop that, the boogeyman will get you!" Others read frightening stories and allow their kids to watch scary movies and terrifying programs on television. (Think of the hideous witch and flying monkey-beasts in *The Wizard of Oz*. And even Sesame Street has a grouchy, growly Cookie Monster.) Finally, parents can inadvertently pass on their own fears. The familiar parent-jumps-on-table-upon-seeing-mouse scenario is a classic example. A child sees this behavior and logically assumes that three-inch gray thing is one awful beast.

Defusing Fear

Of course, a healthy dose of certain fears is more blessing than burden when they keep your child from imminent danger. Consider the handful Dr. Poussaint had as a camp counselor years ago. All summer, several fearless kids collected snake-bites like baseball cards from picking up snakes—by the tail.

In addition, "The recognition of a fear, and the ability of a child to cope with it, can be important learning experiences," Dr. Sarafino notes. "We wonder why kids like watching scary movies. They'll sit there frightened to death, but will keep coming back to watch them. Why? They're proving their bravery just by sitting through it. And, like the theory behind the Greek tragedies, there's a sort of cathartic release going on. This is essentially recognizing and expressing an emotion to overcome it."

But there does come a point with other fears when you only want to stop the scenes, the screaming, or the squeamishness. Many strategies have proved successful. One or a combination of these tactics may help your child conquer the unnecessary fear in his world.

Compassion and patience are *de rigueur* in handling any childhood fear. If they are essential ingredients, communication is the stock.

Regular talks with your child can often get you to the bottom of her fear. Take nightmares, for instance. "Let's say your child has a bad dream, one where she's being chased by something," says Dr. Poussaint. "It's possible she'll view what happened to her in the nightmare as reality—and therefore, something that can happen to her again. This is very common in kids.

"When you talk to her," he says, "ask her what her bad dream was about. Don't only comfort her for having the dream. When she tells you what it was, you have the opportunity to explain about the crazy way dreams work, that all sorts of things happen in the mind that can't happen once we wake up."

Caring conversation can also reveal a problem your child's been harboring. One couple in Hawaii discovered what was lurking behind their three-year-old daughter's new fear of monsters: Two boys in nursery school were terrorizing her.

Couple communication with a little textbook knowledge, and you've got a great way to help prevent fears from turning up in your child.

"Knowing at what age certain fears typically appear is one of the smartest moves you can make," Dr. Sarafino says. "If you know the fear of bugs usually hits during the toddler years, for instance, you can take steps to familiarize your child with insects ahead of time, in a nonthreatening way."

The most common fear to develop in infancy is the fear of separation. Between ages two and six, children develop the greatest number of new fears. The dark, being alone, nightmares, heights, storms and natural disasters, water, imaginary creatures, and animals are typical fears. Older children, while they may still retain one or more of the earlier-appearing fears, may start worrying about school, death, and rejection by peers.

Slaying the Dragons

So now you know the big guns to use when your child is battling a particular fear. Your game plan, though, is just as important.

From "neat little tricks" to general mental attitudes, here are suggestions for helping your child get through (or avoid) five of the most common fears of childhood. These ideas may work with other fears, too.

Darkness ● "This is a very common fear, but probably not universal," says Lawrence Balter, Ph.D., professor of psychology at New York University and host of a nationally syndicated radio talk show. "Some kids hate it. Others can't get to sleep without it." To get your child comfortable when the lights go out, go ahead and use a nightlight, Dr. Balter advises. Just be sure to wean your reluctant sleeper from it gradually. Try moving the light farther from his bed. Cover the bulb for a dimmer glow, or switch to progressively smaller bulbs.

Alison Carivau, of Grand Forks, North Dakota, devised a system to acquaint her two-year-old with being alone in the dark. Whenever he wants a book or toy from his bedroom down the hall, she'll walk with him. The light from the living room gives just enough light to keep the hallway and his room from being totally dark. Her son makes a solo trip when it's time to return the plaything.

Games can also make darkness less scary. Try blind-man's bluff, which challenges your blindfolded child to find and identify several people in a room. Play hide-and-seek with a toy hidden in her dimly-lighted room. Later, try the game with no lights on.

Talking to your child about the dark is important, because chances are it's not just the lack of light that bothers her. Being alone, monsters, "strange" noises and creaks are often interrelated factors that may need to be addressed separately.

You may have been faced with whether to allow refuge in your bed. This is a common give-in among softhearted parents, but experts advise against it. You'll be doing all of you a favor if you gently escort the wayward one back to bed.

Being Alone ● "Every child is afraid of being abandoned," explains Dr. Balter, who is also the author of two books, *Dr. Balter's Child Sense* and *Who's In Control? Dr. Balter's Guide to Discipline without Combat.* "This is often behind the fear of being alone. You need to reassure your child early on that you won't sneak out, and that you'll return when you say you will."

"Give your child some way to channel the energy she's expending on being afraid to something constructive, something fun," adds Jesse Thomas, Ph.D., a marriage, family, and child therapist in La Jolla, California. "Make up a short, special song for her to sing about a brave little child who loved having time all to herself. Or make a present of some drawing paper and crayons. Ask her to draw a picture of your family, and give her tape to hang up her work. This will help her feel like you're not really gone. You could frame a photo of you and your spouse for her to keep with her when you're somewhere else, but making the picture herself will be more comforting.

"Another idea is to leave behind something with the familiar scent of your perfume or after-shave," says Dr. Thomas, who also teaches advanced child therapy at the California School of Professional Psychology. "This is helpful if your child is afraid in the middle of the night, too. One whiff reminds her of the love and protection she gets from you."

Storms ● "We suggest watching storms in amazement," says one mother in Budd Lake, New Jersey. "We taught our son to 'call' to the thunder and to see how beautiful the flashes can be. We also explained how rain makes all the foliage happy and healthy."

"What kids fear most about things like storms is the lack of control they have over it," Dr. Balter says. "The storm is so much bigger and louder than they are." Here's a game to give back the feeling of having at least some control: Get some pots or drums, and several spoons. The only rules are to try to make louder sounds than the thunder and to have fun.

"Another game works well for very young children," notes Dr. Sarafino. "Sit next to a window with your child in your lap. When you both see lightning, say, 'Listen for boom-boom.' When it sounds, say joyously, 'There it is. Oh, boy, that's a good one,' and hug him tightly. If thunder happens and you don't see lightning, joke, 'Ha-ha! They tricked us that time.' Get your child involved, saying 'boom-boom' too."

Funny explanations for thunder ease some kids' fear. One

Pennsylvania couple told tales of angels bowling in heaven and rolling out beer barrels for a party (while the father played "Beer Barrel Polka" on the accordion!). But a simple, scientific explanation can be effective, too, and will also spare you a sheepish confession later. The science lesson can be as basic as, "Clouds bump together and make lightning. Too much water in the air makes rain."

Animals and Insects ● No one's saying you have to help your child make friends with the drooling Doberman down the street. But harmless flies, ants, domestic cats, and their ilk shouldn't be scary.

"Take steps to desensitize your child," says Dr. Balter. "First, draw pictures of the animal or bugs your child fears. Then go to the library together for books on the roles they play in the ecosystem. You might find a natural history museum with an insect collection. Add to these ideas a simple lesson on what to do and what not to do around potentially harmful bees and such, and the fear should ease up."

Monsters and Ghosts ● Robyn Burmood's six-year-old son was never afraid of monsters—"until they were introduced in kindergarten to 'make friends' with them. How ridiculous. He told me, 'When I draw monsters and cut them out, it makes me think they're real.' Well, that's logical! It's a big mistake to say monsters really exist."

Experts are of two minds on this. Those who agree offer an argument like this: If you take your child around his room at night, looking in the closet and under the bed to show the coast is clear, your child will intelligently assume monsters *do* exist (they're just somewhere else at the moment). Otherwise you wouldn't be wasting your time searching.

But, as Dr. Sarafino explains, "It's pretty hard to talk a child out of believing in monsters and ghosts. Especially when he sees and hears about them on television, at the movies, in books, from babysitters and toys and more. The 'evidence' that they're real seems overwhelming."

Sandra Barnes found a way to acknowledge her son Joshua's monster fear without admitting them into existence. "I explained how monsters only live in his imagination," says the Marietta, Georgia, mother. "He now knows *he* has the power to make the monsters scary and mean, or funny and friendly."

Another mother takes a similar approach. "I say, 'Even if they were real, I'm the mommy and I say no monsters are allowed in this house!'"

Dr. Thomas feels the power of parental authority works well. "Your child will believe you when you say, 'we love you so much we would never let anything hurt you.'"

If you'd rather deal directly with your child's monsters, Dr. Thomas suggests having your child draw a picture of a monster and hang it up. "Tell your child, 'Monsters are very afraid of other monsters. If you put this picture where he'll see it, the monster will run away as fast as he can and won't come back.'"

Dr. Balter says that monsters are often a clue some frustrating emotion is bottled up in your child. "Always talk together about the day's events," he says. "Ask what made her happy, sad or angry that day. You may not get immediate results, but you should see the problem's symptoms (the monsters) go away as she opens up."

With any common fear, your goal is to empower your child to handle it sensibly and confidently. If it seems the fear is disrupting his life excessively (interfering with school or socializing, or triggering physical illness, for instance), counseling may be a good idea. Most childhood fears, though, will respond to your caring intervention. And before you know it, the fear will be outgrown like last year's winter coat.

Bone-Building Strategies

Kids may gleefully dress up in skeleton costumes and show off their "bones," only at Halloween, but parents are well aware of that ever-growing skeleton the rest of the year. Pants get too short, shoes get too small (too soon!) and cookies have to be kept higher and higher out of reach. The human skeleton is a lifelong factory of bone-making, but in the years from birth to about age 18, the factory works overtime. And it has to be fed enough of the right raw materials—calcium, phosphorus, vitamins A, C, and D—to keep up with its considerable output.

Baby Bones

The bone factory starts production in the womb, but a newborn's bones are barely half developed. Only a small part of her skeleton is heavily calcified, or hardened—mainly the skull, arms, and legs (which will be bearing her weight soon). The rest is flexible cartilage, much of which becomes harder in her first year. But young bones, like young tree branches, remain somewhat flexible. In fact, one type of bone injury in children, a "greenstick fracture," is actually a severe bend with just a small break on one edge of the bone.

As she gets older, more of your child's bones become calcified through ossification, but the ends of the bone (the epiphyses) remain cartilage. This is the bone's growth zone.

The area between the hardened bone and the cartilage is called the epiphyseal plate. Cartilage cells divide rapidly in a developing child: The cells on the inner side of the epiphyseal plate ossify and add to the length of the bone, while the cells on the joint side of the plate remain cartilage. The result? New jeans every few months.

This process continues for about 18 years in girls and 20 years in boys. Growth stops when the epiphyses become bone, leaving cartilage only at the jointed ends. Mercifully for parents, the last bones to stop growing have nothing to do with designer jeans or fashionable sneakers. They are the collar bones.

Feeding the Skeleton

Your child is growing the skeleton that will have to support her the rest of her life. So nurturing strong bones isn't just a matter of ensuring normal development. Feeding her well and teaching her good diet and exercise habits now will give her the framework for healthy adulthood.

The growth of healthy bones depends on adequate supplies of several nutrients. First on the list of requirements are calcium and phosphorus, the minerals which form the actual bone. Ninety-nine percent of the body's calcium is stored in the skeleton, but some is always circulating in the blood and cellular fluid. Calcium is essential for nerve function, for blood coagulation, muscle movement and the heart, as well as the bones. If enough is not available for these vital needs from the diet, the body takes it out of its savings account—the skeleton.

Phosphorus and fluoride are also essential for bone growth and development, as are several vitamins of whose roles in bone growth you might not be aware. Without vitamin A, bone remodeling—the constant breakdown and re-creation of bone cells—is impaired. Vitamin C is needed for the formation of collagen. Collagen creates the foundation on which calcium is laid.

Vitamin D, called the "sunshine" vitamin because ultraviolet light triggers its production in the body, plays several complex parts in building bone. First of all, it aids absorption of dietary calcium in the intestines and phosphorus in the kidneys. It is also essential to making calcium available to bone cells.

Lack of vitamin D causes rickets, a disease in which a child's bones do not calcify but remain soft, resulting in poor growth and deformities of the legs, rib cage, pelvis and skull. It can cause death in young children. Rickets is rare now in the Western world, but it was tragically common in Britain and America in the 17th to early 20th centuries. With increased industrialization, cities became mazes of dim alleys between tall buildings. Ferocious coal-smoke pollution darkened city skies. What sun shone between buildings had little chance to filter through the smog; and among the poor and working classes, city dwellers were often working inside for long hours anyway, with no chance to be outdoors. This congested city setting led to widespread vitamin D deficiency—and to generations of people who were short, sickly, and bowlegged. Upper-class kids, who generally lived outside city limits, had a lower incidence of vitamin D deficiency.

The only time American doctors see a case of vitamin D deficiency-rickets nowadays is in children who are being exclusively breastfed after about nine months or those raised on a strict vegan diet, which excludes all animal foods, even dairy. We've gone from being sun shunners to sun worshippers in less than a century, which pretty much ensures that kids build up sufficient vitamin D reserves. Since vitamin D is oil-soluble, the body can store a summer's worth of sunshine in body fat for use in the dark days of winter. Kids' other major source of vitamin D is milk.

"Bone" Appétit

It's not just dairy industry hype—milk really is just about a perfect food as far as bones are concerned. Calories, calcium, vitamin A, protein: Almost every nutrient growing bones (or mature ones, for that matter) need is in milk. Milk got even closer to perfection when dairies began adding vitamin D in the 1930s. No wonder pediatricians and childhood nutrition experts put milk on the top of kids' menus.

But milk has been the cause of many a dinner-table wrangle. "No dessert until you drink your milk" is probably one of the most common phrases spoken in American households. Lots of kids don't like milk—at least not in a glass. (Ice cream is another story.) And for some kids, milk equals misery, because they lack a milk-sugar digesting intestinal enzyme called lactase. For these lactose-intolerant people, milk packs a bloated, crampy, gassy punch.

"If your child won't or can't drink milk, let her eat it instead," suggests Jo-Anne Heslin, a registered dietitian who is an expert in children's nutrition at Adelphi University on Long Island. "Cheese, pudding, custard, and yogurt are all big favorites with kids and are a painless way of getting milk into them." Heslin explains that either heating or fermenting milk alters the sugars so lactose-intolerant children can digest it. And most of the lactase is pressed out of hard cheeses in the liquid part of milk, called whey.

"Don't make a big issue out of drinking milk," says Heslin. "Just find other calcium-rich—and that means dairy—foods your child will eat instead."

Parents of lactose-intolerant children have lots of options these days, notes Heslin. "Many local dairies make low-lactose milk, cheeses, and ice cream," she says.

The Lactaid Company in New Jersey not only sells dairy

products with the enzyme added to aid digestion, it now markets the substance in liquid and tablet form. You can add the liquid to your child's milk, or give her a tablet or two before she eats ice cream. The Lactaid company will send you free samples of both their liquid and tablets if you call (800) 257-8650 during East Coast business hours (in New Jersey, call 609-645-7500).

One final tip: If milk makes your child miserable, try cutting down the serving size, suggests Heslin. "Lots of kids who get stomachaches and the rest of the intolerance symptoms from eight ounces of milk can handle three or four ounces with no problems."

As for the issue of whole versus 2 percent or skim milk, Heslin believes you should not switch a child to a lower fat milk before age two. "Milk is a very important source of calories for small children. After age two, I think 2 percent milk is best for the whole family," she says.

These days calcium-fortified foods like cereal and orange juice are available, too, and there are other good natural sources of calcium. But, as Heslin notes wryly, "Greens, tofu, and fish are not big favorites with kids. It's a good idea to get them to eat a variety of foods, but the chief source of nutrients for their bones is going to be dairy foods."

What about calcium tablets, the chic supplement of the 1980s? "I use them in my practice only as a last resort," Heslin reports, "and I always emphasize that they are a *supplement*, not a substitute for calcium in the diet."

Get Those Bones Moving

Even an adequate intake of calcium can't ensure strong bones if those bones don't see some action. In a study at the University of Utah, doctors found that kids who were big TV watchers and didn't get much exercise had lower bone mineral content (BMC) than kids who walked, biked, and generally got a lot of exercise. This happened even though all the kids were getting adequate calcium in their diets.

"There is no danger in a slightly lower BMC for children," says Gary M. Chan, M.D., an associate professor of pediatrics at the university. "We aren't seeing bone problems in healthy children, but we are concerned that the lower bone mineral content will be carried into adulthood and result in bone problems then. My recommendations for children are simply to get good nutrition and be active."

And being active means more than getting involved in organized sports. In fact, New Orleans pediatrician George Sterne, M.D., believes contact sports are not for grade schoolers. "Their bodies just aren't developed enough to take the knocks. Competitive sports like running, swimming or well-supervised Little League are okay, provided it's what the child wants to do. The things to emphasize are walking, biking, swimming— activities a child can carry over into adult life. These are the kinds of exercises you can do as a family, too," he says.

Outdoor exercise is a good way to build up vitamin D reserves as well. "Casual exposure to the sun is the biggest source of vitamin D for anyone who drinks fewer than four glasses of milk a day," says Michael Holick, M.D., Ph.D., chief of the endocrine unit at Boston City Hospital and one of the foremost American experts on vitamin D. "Other dairy foods don't have any D, and other than fish and fish oils, there are no other food sources of it."

Recently Dr. Holick and colleague Ann Webb, Ph.D. discovered that the winter sun in Boston has no vitamin D-triggering power at all. "It seems that the further north you go, the longer the time that you get no vitamin D from the sun becomes," he says. "In Boston, the period lasts from November to March. On the other hand, in sunny southern cities like Los Angeles, the sun lets the body synthesize vitamin D all year long. We're not at all sure at this point, but we speculate that somewhere around the latitude of Virginia you begin to lose this year-round power of the sun."

Dr. Holick also discovered that a sunscreen with an SPF as low as eight is enough to cut off vitamin D production in the skin. But he says not to worry that you are starving your child's skeleton while protecting his skin from sun damage. "No parent can manage to cover the whole kid with sunscreen. Any little gap in coverage is enough to allow adequate sunshine to reach the skin."

THOSE ARE THE BREAKS

Kids' bones are much more flexible than adults', but they will bend only so far. Even babies, who seem as agile as eels, can break bones. Prevention is best, so try fallproofing your house with stair gates. Get down on your toddler's eye level and look for things that might be fun to climb up on or pull over. Remove temptation wherever you see it. Still, accidents will happen, so it is a good idea to learn how to recognize and handle a childhood fracture.

A broken bone *hurts*. In fact, a child with a fracture may be crying too hard to tell you what happened or where it hurts. So you may have to look for loss of normal function. A broken limb doesn't work—a leg won't hold weight, an arm can't be raised. The muscles around a fracture are rigid. Hard, tense muscles are a natural splint. Finally, the area near the break is swollen and bruised. This is due to tissue and muscle damage caused by the bone's movement.

If you think your child has broken a bone, call your doctor at once. Do not attempt to move a child who may have a spine or neck injury—call an ambulance. Do not let the child put any weight on a suspected leg, ankle or foot fracture. Immobilize a broken arm by wrapping a large towel around the child's upper body and arm, with the elbow just slightly bent. Be especially careful if you think the upper arm is broken. Excessive movement risks severing the arm's main artery.

With proper medical attention, children's bones mend quickly. The same process that makes them grow upwards so fast knits them back together quickly, too. Most likely, your child will be over her accident long before you are.

Fast Action
for Outdoor Ills and Spills

When we look back on our own childhood summers, we tend to remember finding new ways to get into trouble, vaulting through fields of wildflowers, cheeks colored by the sun and high spirits, bouncing off in cars packed with vacation gear, dolphining through pools, ponds, and waves, cycling off to the adventures only summertime offers.

But, as our parents before us, we now see summer's flip side: chipped teeth from bike wrecks, bedsheets stuck to backs of sun-seared thighs, crazed itching from poison ivy, oak, or sumac, stopping a dozen times on the way to the beach for a car-sick child, maybe even the frightening near loss of a young child's playmate who never learned to swim but wouldn't be left out of the fun.

"Any parent who has raised two or three kids has probably learned as much about basic first aid as a medical school graduate," says Kenneth S. Gray, M.D., certified emergency physician and medical director of Doctors Care Medical Center in San Diego.

Most outdoor ills require nothing more than a kiss and some judicious home remedies. But, if in doubt, says Dr. Gray, let a doctor check it out.

Cuts and Scrapes

When your child comes home bleeding, instead of reaching for the bottle of hydrogen peroxide, turn on the tap water. "A wound can be cleaned with water only," says Dr. Gray. "Chemicals are not necessary. Just rinse it out thoroughly and put a clean bandage on it to protect it."

If the skin has been cut, you can wipe off any obvious debris, like gravel or grass, but don't try to clean down into the cut itself. Control bleeding by pressing down right on the wound. "Cuts usually don't hurt much at first," says Dr. Gray, "so you can apply pressure without hurting your child. A tourniquet is not a good idea." If the bleeding has not stopped after about 15 minutes, see a doctor. It could need stitching.

Some parents like to use a topical antibacterial ointment to prevent infection. "It's not usually necessary if you've washed off the wound well," says Dr. Gray, "but an ointment will keep the bandage from sticking to the skin while it's healing." Check the label of multiple-antibiotic creams first, though, to be sure your child is not allergic to one of the components. Some people are sensitive to neomycin, an ingredient in some ointments. A certain degree of redness is a normal part of the healing process. But if the skin around the scrape becomes more red, hot and tender, it may be infected. See your doctor for further treatment.

Poisonous Plant Rashes

If you know your child has been exposed to poison ivy, oak, or sumac, try to get to soap and water fast. The plant oils may be on her clothing and shoes, so remove them carefully and wash them as soon as you can. Scrubbing her skin within 30 minutes of contact may prevent the eruption of a rash; sensitive children should wash within five minutes of exposure. And don't forget to scrub under fingernails, where hiding plant oils can spread the rash every time the child scratches. In spite of what you might have heard, fluid that oozes from the rash *cannot* spread it, either to other children or to other parts of your child's body.

Over-the-counter oral diphenhydramine hydrochloride, such as Benadryl elixir or tablets, helps ease itching and can be given to "any child old enough to run around in poisonous plants," says Dr. Gray. Cool baths and compresses and drying lotions will make your child more comfortable, but nothing will stop the progress of the rash. Hot showers and getting overheated won't worsen the rash but will make it itch more. The goal is to stop the scratching and so prevent skin infections from developing.

If you suspect poisonous plants are being burned (in a brush pile, for example), keep your child away from the area. The oils can be carried with the smoke for long distances.

Insect Bites and Stings

A number of insects may hitch a ride on your child's skin when she's playing outdoors. Most cause minor discomforts that you can treat with common household items.

Mosquitoes ● Cool compresses can help bring down swelling and relieve some itching. Benadryl also helps.

Ticks ● Don't try to pull the tick off. A part of the insect could stay lodged in the skin and start an infection. Use a burnt match or alcohol to irritate the tick and make it withdraw from the skin by itself. If these procedures fail, have your pediatrician remove the tick.

Stinging Insects ● Cold compresses and an oral antihistamine offer the best relief.

Parents should also know the symptoms of a bee sting allergy: Hives all over the body, chest tightness, hoarseness, wheezing, swollen tongue or face, dizziness, fainting, or shock. Severe reactions to bee stings can be fatal, so get your child to a doctor fast.

Sunburn

Evidence keeps piling up that children who fry now will pay later. Researchers say up to three-fourths of skin cancer can be prevented by regular sunscreen use during the first 18 years of life. Protect your child's skin by routinely applying sunscreen whenever she plays outside.

Most sunburns are first-degree burns. Cool compresses and mild pain relievers, such as aspirin or acetaminophen, will help relieve the pain and burning. (Aspirin is especially useful for reducing swelling.) Don't use ice, which can damage burned skin. All other remedies—skin creams, aloe vera, butter, even mayonnaise—are not necessary, according to Dr. Gray.

If your child's skin is blistering, she has suffered a second-degree burn. The treatment is the same, but if more than a small area is affected, you should have her treated by a doctor.

Any sunburn in a child under one year old should be treated by a doctor.

Swimmer's Ear

Children who turn into fish during summer are prone to developing infections in their outer ears. Wax that normally lines and protects the ear canal washes away after too much dunking, leaving the skin open to infection. The main symptom of swimmer's ear is pain that gets worse when you pull on the earlobe. "Patients often tell me they can't lie on that ear," says Dr. Gray. You may be able to see redness and swelling if the infection has spread to the outer ear. Your doctor can prescribe appropriate treatment.

Rest assured that swimmer's ear won't lead to hearing loss, because the inner ear is protected by the ear drum. But there have been cases of infection spreading to outer-ear cartilage and causing "cauliflower ear" when it's left untreated.

The best treatment is preventive, says Dr. Gray. Use one of the alcohol and boric acid solutions sold for that purpose in any drugstore. Put a few drops in each ear whenever your child's been in the water for awhile. Ear plugs usually don't help; they often just trap water inside the ear. Don't use preventive drops after the ear has already become infected, advises Dr. Gray. This will hurt, making your child more fearful the next time. Besides, the drops only prevent infections; they won't cure them.

Submersion

Everyone knows that the only response to a drowning accident is to call 911 for emergency medical help. If someone trained in first aid is on hand, mouth-to-mouth resuscitation should be administered to a child who has stopped breathing, and full CPR if the heartbeat has stopped.

What many people don't realize is that any case of submersion should be evaluated by a doctor. Your child may have been pulled from the water before she lost consciousness, but she may have suffered an injury that could later cause serious illness, so get prompt medical attention. "In any near-drowning accident," says Dr. Gray, "even if the child is awake and alert, we will keep her overnight to make sure there are no delayed breathing problems."

Heat Illness

Infants left in cars and kids playing summertime football are heat's favorite victims. Parents can help by never leaving a baby in a car and by making sure adolescent athletes drink enough liquids before and during hot weather exercise.

Heat illness comes in two forms: heat exhaustion and heatstroke. In heat exhaustion, your child's temperature may stay normal, but her skin will be clammy and she'll seem tired, headachy, dizzy or nauseated. Get her to a cool spot, remove her clothes, cover her with towels cooled in ice water and have her checked by a doctor.

Heatstroke can be fatal and requires immediate medical help. Look for a rise in body temperature to 105°F or higher, and skin that's hot, red and dry. Your child may even lose consciousness. On the way to the doctor, remove her clothes and cover her with ice water-soaked towels. Fast action in a case of heatstroke may save your child's life.

Knocked-Out Tooth

Rough-and-tumble childhood play may cause a tooth to tumble right out of your child's mouth. Don't panic; if you get the child and the tooth to a dentist fast, chances are the tooth can be saved.

If the tooth is dirty, grasp it by the crown, not the roots, and rinse it gently in cool running water. Don't scrub it. Try to put the tooth back into its socket, provided your child is calm enough. If you can't, put it in a cup of milk or water or wrap it in a clean, damp cloth to transport it to the dentist. Teeth that are replaced in the mouth by a dentist within 30 minutes after the injury have a chance of becoming reattached and functioning normally.

Car or Bike Accident

Children's chances of accidental injury go up during the more active days of summer. "There are a few basic things to remember when your child is involved in an accident," says Dr. Gray. "If she's been hit by car or fallen from a bike or skateboard —whenever there is a large mass colliding with your child or great speed involved—there's the potential for severe injury. You must get emergency medical care. Don't even try to move her, unless she is lying in a spot where she is in danger of being further injured."

If you are the only person on hand, see what you can do, then go get help. Before you even touch the child, talk to her. Asking "Are you all right?" or "Where does it hurt?" will help you determine what is wrong before you do something that could worsen an injury.

"The first person on the scene should try to remember the details of the accident," says Dr. Gray. "How was the child lying when you found her? Was she bleeding? Was she breathing? Were her eyes open? Was she talking? Was she moving spontaneously or was she limp? That information will help the medical personnel decide how to help her.

"Crowd control will be hard," says Dr. Gray, who has seen his share of accidents. "People crowd around and shout out a lot of things they think will help. If you want to be effective, the important thing is to keep your cool."

Head Injury

Whenever you suspect your child has had a head injury, remember to protect her neck also. "People just worry about whether the child is conscious," says Dr. Gray. "But she could be unconscious *and* have a broken neck. If she is moved, the spinal cord can be injured, with permanent damage to the nervous system."

Remember that any loss of consciousness should be medically evaluated. If your child gets a bump on the head, has a momentary blackout and recovers, she should be seen by a doctor.

Even if a child with a head injury does not lose consciousness, there are other symptoms to watch for: persistent nausea and vomiting, visual changes such as blurriness or double vision, persistent headache, a large lump on the head that continues to get larger, or any inappropriate behavior like loss of memory about the accident. "All of these could mean brain injury," says Dr. Gray. "It might be just a concussion, but it could indicate something more serious. The appearance of any of these symptoms should be evaluated by a doctor."

Many head injuries can be avoided by wearing a helmet while bike riding or skateboarding, notes Dr. Gray. A helmet cushions the head in a fall and protects it from sharp objects.

Broken Bones

Naturally, a quick trip to the doctor is in order if you suspect a broken bone, but you may have to splint the bone before you can move the child. If you do, support the limb as it is, don't try to straighten it. "If an arm or leg is severely bent, people want to try to straighten it," says Dr. Gray. "It's a gut-wrenching experience for the layperson to see a fracture like that. But you may cause injury to blood vessels and nerves when they move against the edge of bone. Just try to immobilize the limb in the position you find it."

The same rules about immobilization apply when there is an "open fracture" (meaning the skin has been torn open over the site of a broken bone). But no matter how bad the flesh wound looks, don't try to wash it out. Wipe away any large debris like grass or gravel that might be around the wound. Put a clean cloth over the break and get medical care as soon as possible.

Sprained Wrist or Ankle

Sprains are common hazards of sports. Most sprains can be treated by elevating the limb and applying ice packs, followed by resting the affected part. Sometimes it's hard for a layperson to tell a sprain from a broken bone, and a bad sprain requires medical treatment as much as a break. The rule of thumb, according to Dr. Gray: If your child can't use her arm, or can't walk on her leg, if the pain is severe or seems to be getting worse instead of better, it's time to see a doctor.

CHILDREN'S INJURY INDEX

Below are statistics on the annual toll that accidents take on our children.

- Accidents—including drownings, falls, and auto accidents—are the largest cause of death for kids aged 1 to 14 years.
- 8,800 children under the age of 15 were injured during one particular year in accidents involving lawn mowers.
- During strenuous exercise, 85°F is the danger zone in young athletes for heatstroke when the relative humidity is at 50 percent, but it drops to 60° at 100 percent humidity.
- 29 percent of all eye injuries happen to children younger than 11 years. 78 percent of the victims are boys.
- More than 6,000 sports-related eye injuries happen to children aged 5 to 14, usually while playing baseball.
- 140,000 children aged 5 to 14 were treated for baseball-related injuries in emergency rooms during one two-year period.
- 400,000 children are treated in emergency rooms for bike injuries each year. Up to 600 children die each year in bike accidents.
- 55 percent of bike injuries occur during daylight hours.
- 44 percent of bike accidents are caused by children losing control of their bikes, compared to only 17 percent caused by collisions with automobiles.
- 11,000 children a year are killed by cars.
- 200,000 injuries involving playground equipment are serious enough to require emergency room treatment each year.
- 40 percent of drownings happen to children under age 11.
- 3,000 children under age five suffer near-drowning each year; one third of these are left with brain injuries.
- 68 percent of near-drownings take place during a momentary lapse of attention in a parent who is supervising the child.
- 13,000 children between 5 and 15 are injured when diving or using pool slides.

Vaporize with Caution

Remember having a cold when you were a kid? Tucked into a warm bed, Vicks VapoRub smeared on your chest, drowsing off to the comforting burble and hiss of the hot-steam vaporizer. You couldn't help but feel better.

But while the vaporizer may have helped you *feel* better, it had nothing to do with helping you *get* better.

"There is absolutely no evidence that vaporizers have any therapeutic benefit in upper respiratory illnesses other than croup," says pediatric pulmonary specialist Robert L. Hopkins, M.D., of the Tulane University School of Medicine in New Orleans. "Adding humidity may make a child with a cold a bit more comfortable, but it's not going to make him get better any faster."

That may sound like heresy, but Dr. Hopkins isn't a renegade or a medical revolutionary. Even though it seems every baby and child care book says to turn on the vaporizer at the first sign of a sniffle, none of the doctors we interviewed believes they have any real effect on colds or stuffy noses. The way to help clear congestion, they say, is by adding moisture internally—the old standard advice to "drink plenty of fluids."

So what about vaporizers? They still have their uses. But the valid uses may just be different than you think. Dr. Hopkins points out that the water droplets produced by standard vaporizers, whether the steam or cool-mist type, are simply too big to reach any further than the nose or throat. That helps keep nasal passages moist, and less likely to bleed, but it doesn't have much, if anything, to do with helping a child with a cold breathe easier, which is just what most parents are trying to do with a vaporizer.

While vaporizers won't cure (or prevent) a cold, they *will* help croup—the barking cough and whistling, noisy breathing that has frightened generations of new parents. Moisture will open a croup-closed throat. The time-honored way of dealing with a croupy child is to take him into the bathroom and run the tub or shower until the room is like a steam bath. But a vaporizer will keep the humidity high long after your hot water runs out. Our experts agreed that your doctor would be right to recommend a vaporizer for croup.

Many Ways to Make Mist

It used to be easy to choose a vaporizer—there was only one kind! Now there's a bewildering array of vaporizers on the market. How do you know which type is right for your child?

You can still find the hot-steam variety, but most doctors believe they are too risky, especially around small children. "Would you put a saucepan of boiling water next to a two-year-old?" asks Dr. Hopkins. In 1979, he and two colleagues at Tulane treated three children for steam burns caused by hot-water vaporizers. They noted that over 600 such injuries are reported each year, but many more accidents like these probably occur.

Cool-mist vaporizers are safer; but as pediatrician George Sterne, M.D., points out, "You have to be fanatical about keeping them clean. Bacteria and molds grow in water, and if a unit isn't kept scrupulously clean, you wind up throwing germs and mold into the air along with the moisture. That can cause infections and allergy problems."

With the arrival of ultrasonic room humidifiers, the formerly homely vaporizer actually became high-tech. While the old-style units work either by turning water to steam or by throwing droplets into the air under pressure, the ultrasonics rely on a tiny electronic "transducer" that vibrates water into a fine mist. The transducer is the reason the ultrasonics are so much more expensive ($50 to $140, compared to $10 to $30 for the conventional kind), although as more electronics companies now make them, prices have dropped somewhat. The ultrasonics have been touted as optimal humidification—silent, where conventional room humidifiers are annoyingly noisy, and hypoallergenic, since the vibration shatters molds and microbes in the water into tiny bits too small to cause problems. (The latter claim appears to be true. *Consumer Reports* found that ultrasonics would probably not cause problems unless a person was already sensitive to molds.)

But the biggest difference between ultrasonic vaporizers and the conventional ones, and the one which concerns many doctors, is the size of the water particles they put out. Droplets from an ultrasonic are so tiny they can actually penetrate the respiratory system right down to the lungs. That's not necessarily a good thing.

"With the ultrasonics, you run the risk of piling water on top of the secretions already congested in a child's lungs," Dr. Sterne warns. "You don't want fluid there; that can lead to pneumonia. What you do want is to get the fluid *under* the congestion, so to speak, by drinking water and juices. I'm not saying using an ultrasonic vaporizer is going to cause pneumonia every time. But you have to use some sense, especially with a small child. Don't shut him up in a room with the unit running; keep the door of the bedroom open. And most definitely don't use one of these if your doctor says to build a tent around the child's bed and vaporizer, which is sometimes necessary with croup."

A Mania for Moisture

It seems like we develop a mania for moisture in the winter. It's true that a closed-up, heated house can become uncomfortably dry. Static sparks fly when you walk across a rug or give a pussycat a friendly pat. Your skin and throat get parched. But resist the urge to transform your home into a rain forest. There is such a thing as too much humidity.

"The normal human respiratory tract does very well in quite dry air," maintains William R. Solomon, M.D., chief of the Allergy Division at the University of Michigan Medical Center. "The concept many people have—that low humidity is *definitely* harmful—is mistaken."

As an allergist, Dr. Solomon is especially concerned about the irritants that thrive in a moist climate. "Even people who don't have a mold allergy may develop one if they have a humidifier that's spraying the stuff around. There's a real possibility that the yeast and mold could sensitize the person and they'd wind up developing new symptoms because of the humidifier," he says.

Dr. Solomon and Dr. Sterne agree that a daily scrubbing is essential if you do choose to use a vaporizer. "Scour all the inside surfaces thoroughly with something rough, such as a plastic pot scrubber, and rinse the unit carefully," Dr. Solomon says. And he warns that chemical cleaners are not only unnecessary, but may also be dangerous. "You don't want to put anything in the water that could possibly be toxic," he cautions. "If you spray some of these 'mold preventives' into the air, there's a real possibility of causing a skin reaction as well."

Beware also of advice to use bleach to kill what's living in the humidifier. Dr. Solomon warns that respiratory irritation could result. There's no shortcut to vaporizer cleanliness. "Elbow grease is the answer," says Dr. Solomon.

How Much Moisture?

"Almost no one is going to be harmed by a relative humidity factor of around 20 to 25 percent," says Dr. Solomon.

Keep that in mind if you decide to buy a vaporizer or humidifier. Look for one that shuts itself off when the humidity reaches a certain point. Such units have a "humidistat," which automatically cycles the machine on and off to maintain the desired humidity. You're most likely to find this feature on the ultrasonics, although some cool-mist vaporizers have humidistats, too.

Before you buy, check how easily a unit can be cleaned. Can you reach into the water reservoir easily? Can the vents and the parts which draw up the water be cleaned with a brush? Does a brush come with the unit, or must you buy one separately?

If your child seems to be more comfortable when you use a vaporizer, use it only at night. A pot of water on the stove or set on a radiator may be all the moisture you need during the day. And don't forget house plants; their green color will remind you of summer while they breathe moist oxygen into your home.

Index

Rodale Press, Inc., publishes PREVENTION, America's leading health magazine.
For information on how to order your subscription,
write to PREVENTION, Emmaus, PA 18098.